GW01564091

A Pocket Guide to

LOVING
Sex

A Pocket Guide to

LOVING SEX

HEADLINE

Copyright © 1995, 1996, 1997 Marshall Cavendish Ltd

This edition published in 1997 by
HEADLINE BOOK PUBLISHING

10 9 8 7 6 5 4 3 2

Produced by Marshall Cavendish Books, London
(a division of Marshall Cavendish Partworks, Ltd)

All illustrations courtesy of MC Picture Library
The right of Jane Hertford to be identified as the Author of the Work has
been asserted by her in accordance with the Copyright, Designs and
Patents Act 1988

All rights reserved. No part of this publication may be reproduced, stored in a
retrieval system or transmitted in any form or by any means electronic, mechanical,
photocopying, recording or otherwise, without the prior written permission of the
publisher and the copyright holder, nor be otherwise circulated in any form of binding
or cover other than that in which it is published and without a similar condition being
imposed on the subsequent purchaser.

Senior Editor: Sarah Bloxham
Editorial Consultant: Krystyna Zukowska
Senior Art Editor: Joyce Mason
Designer: Richard Newport
Picture Researcher: Marcia Mullings
Production Controller: Craig Chubb

Library of Congress Cataloging-in-Publication Data:
Hertford, Jane
Pocket Guide to Loving Sex
1. Title
613.96

ISBN 0 7472 1648 7

Printed and bound in Italy

HEADLINE BOOK PUBLISHING
A division of Hodder Headline PLC
338 Euston Road, London NW1 3BH

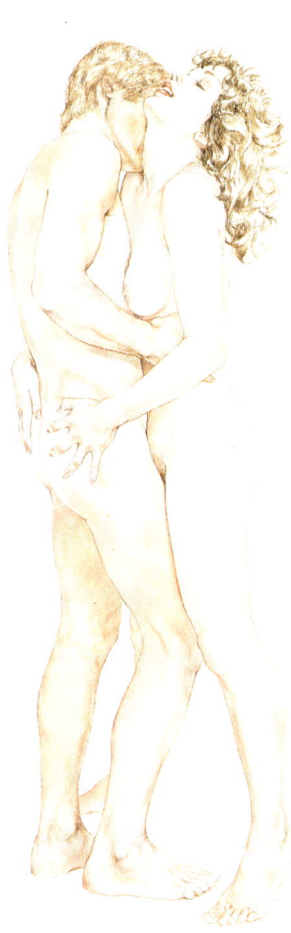

Contents

chapter one
What It's All About
9

chapter two
Setting the Scene
17

chapter three
Foreplay
27

chapter four
Positions & Performance
51

chapter five
Games & Erotic Toys
79

chapter six
Afterplay
91

Index and
Acknowledgements
96

A POCKET GUIDE TO LOVING SEX

There are now so many books available on the market telling us how to get into various sexual positions, each increasing in athleticism and improbability, that very often we forget that making love is something to be enjoyed and cherished by two people.

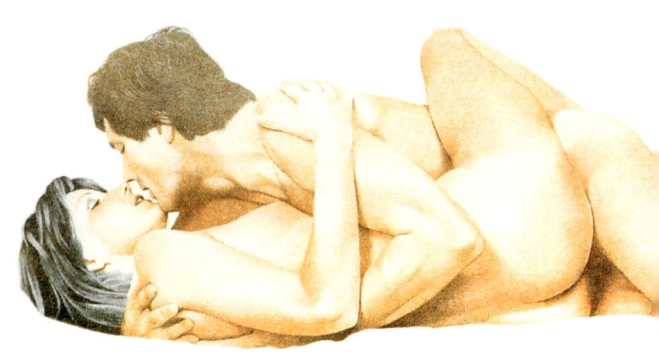

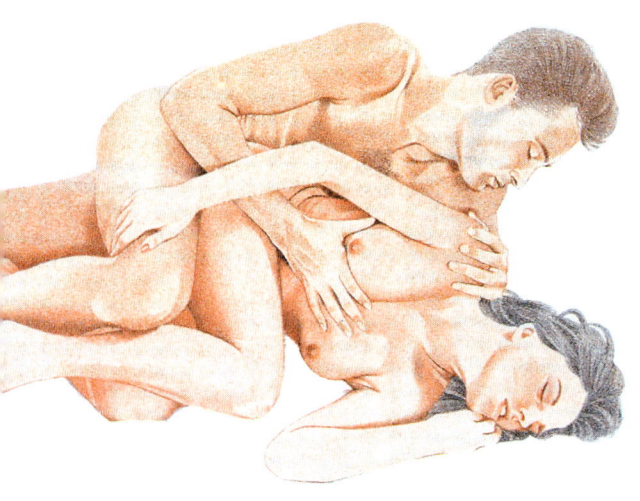

Making love isn't simply a vehicle for the demonstration of an individual's sexual prowess. Sex is the culmination of the bond between a couple and lovemaking starts a long time before reaching the bedroom door. You must remember that making love begins in the mind: you must respect your partner to really enjoy sex. And learning how to become

a considerate and sensitive lover is just the first step towards the two of you gaining sexual satisfaction and fulfilment. This handy pocket book shows you how you can go about achieving this.

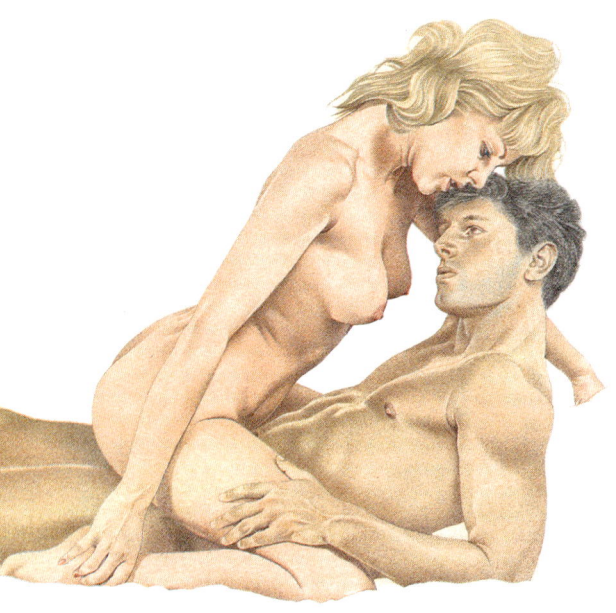

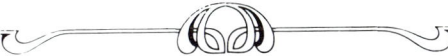

chapter one

WHAT IT'S ALL ABOUT

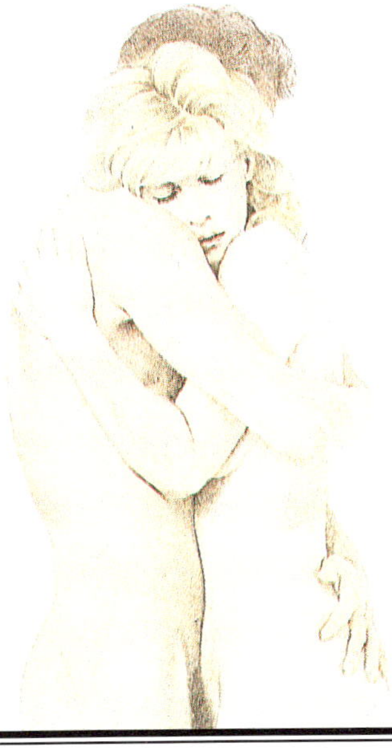

SEX AND 'SEXERCISE'

Good sex requires energy and plenty of stamina. You'll enjoy a far more satisfying sex life if you are healthy and basically fit. That means eating the right things and exercising regularly.

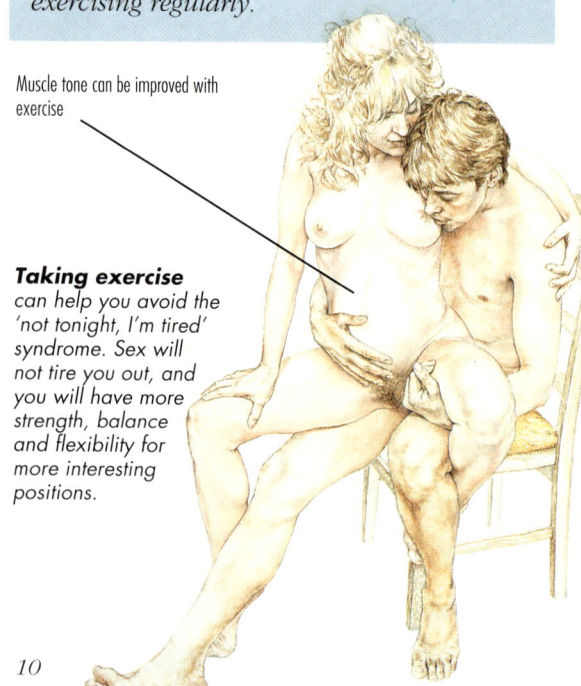

Muscle tone can be improved with exercise

Taking exercise can help you avoid the 'not tonight, I'm tired' syndrome. Sex will not tire you out, and you will have more strength, balance and flexibility for more interesting positions.

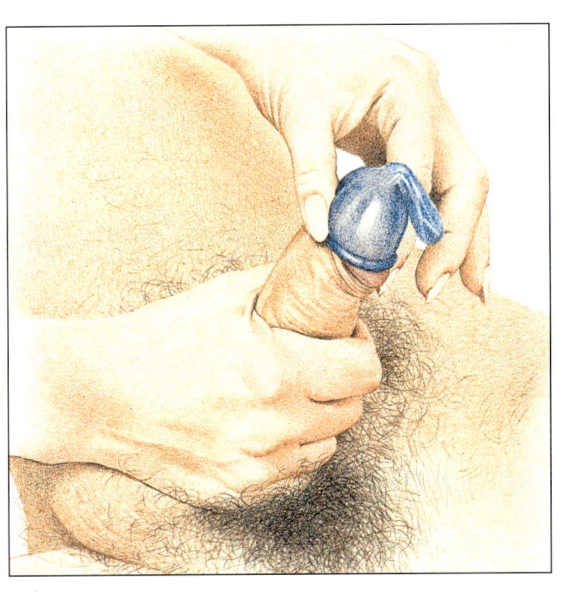

Keeping your body healthy also extends to keeping it free from infection. Using barrier methods of contraception, such as condoms, can prevent the spread of sexually transmitted diseases (STDs) and the HIV virus.

To put on a condom, place the unrolled condom on the top of the erect penis, squeezing out any air from the tip with your thumb and forefinger and pushing back the foreskin. Hold the base of the penis in one hand and unroll the condom over it with the other.

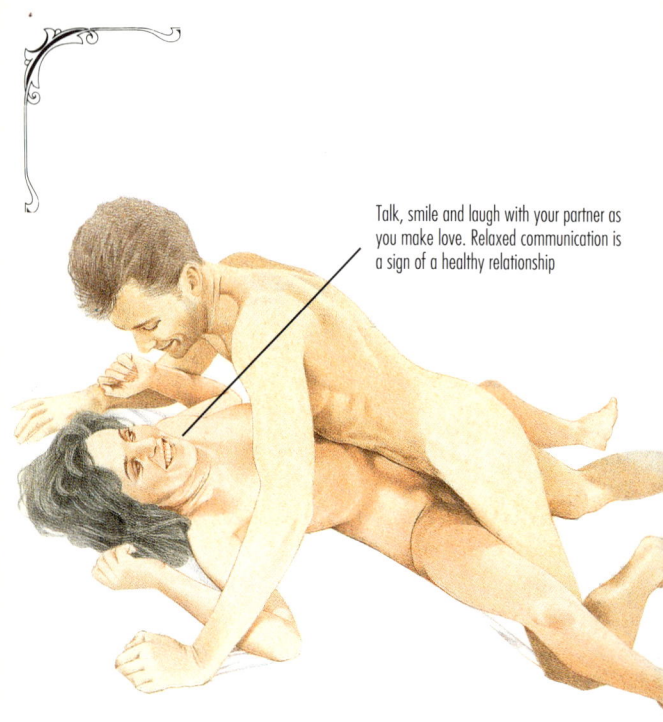

Talk, smile and laugh with your partner as you make love. Relaxed communication is a sign of a healthy relationship

Self-confidence in your appearance is an added benefit of exercise and good eating. Feeling secure with your body is not only liberating sexually, it also makes you more desirable to your partner.

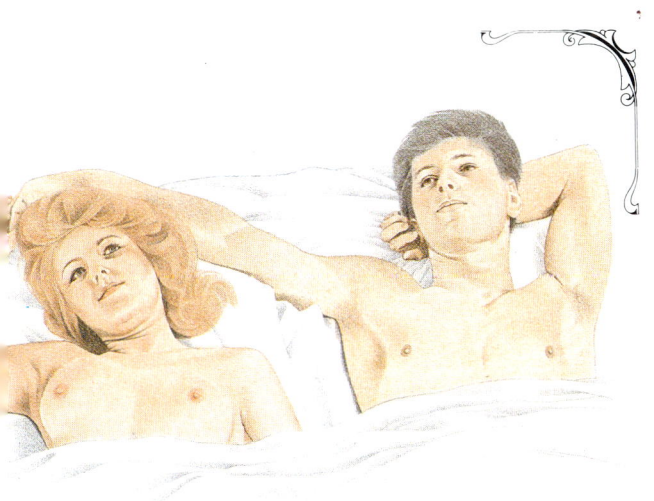

Sexual intercourse is not the be all and end all of making love. Sometimes penetration may not be a preferred option. Perhaps illness, menstruation or an advanced stage of pregnancy (or just after childbirth) makes it difficult; perhaps a partner is not free from STDs or the HIV virus. In other cases, sexual intimacy may be desired but, due to medication, fatigue, stress or other factors, getting and keeping an erection is difficult.

There are other ways of having satisfying and loving sex. Oral sex (with a condom, if either of you is infected) or using vibrators is also pleasurable, as is mutual caressing, hugging and massaging. Just lying in bed having an intimate conversation and sharing your sexual fantasies can also be highly erotic.

ORGASMS

The sexual response of each sex differs. Her climax takes longer to achieve than his, but may last longer, and she can more easily have multiple orgasms. He tends to climax more quickly, more inevitably, and with less stimulation.

Female orgasm
Along with body caresses, special attention should be paid to a woman's labia and clitoris, building stimulation with steady rhythm. As she becomes aroused, the vagina lengthens and becomes lubricated and the labia enlarge; the breasts swell and the nipples become erect. With continued stimulation, sexual tension gradually intensifies until it is released in a series of pleasurable contractions.

Male orgasm
As a man becomes aroused, blood flows into the penis and is trapped, causing it to become erect. As he penetrates his partner and starts to thrust, his sexual tension intensifies quickly. It is released in a series of contractions by the muscles in and around the penis and by the ejaculation of semen from the penis.

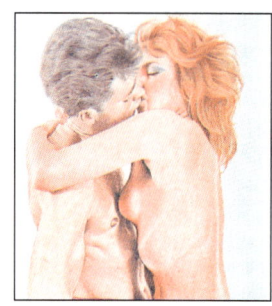

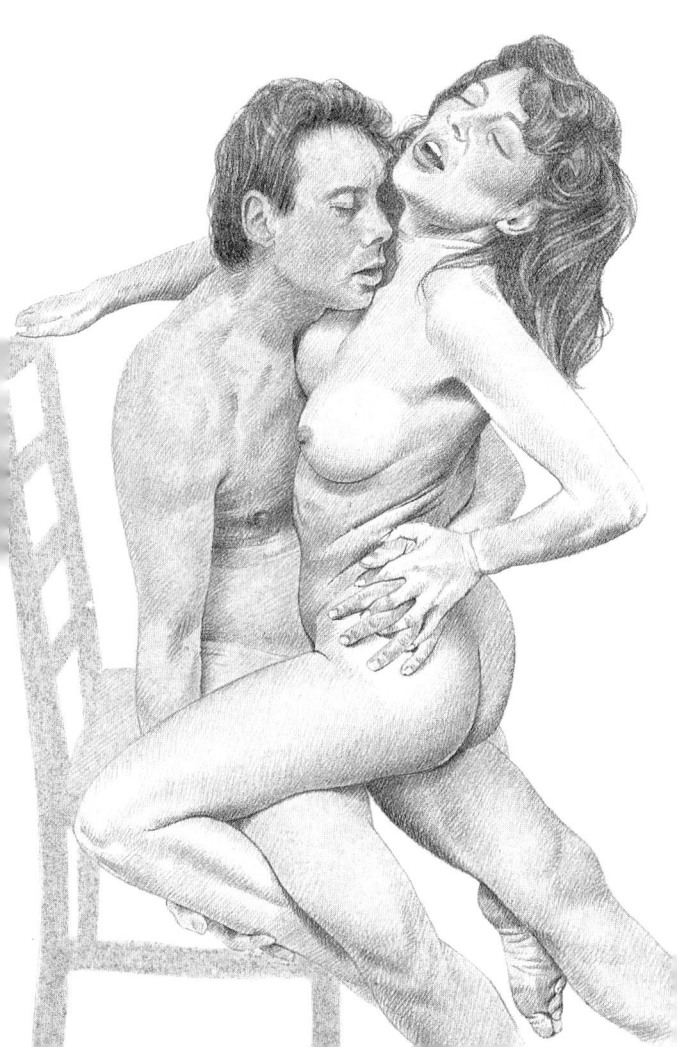

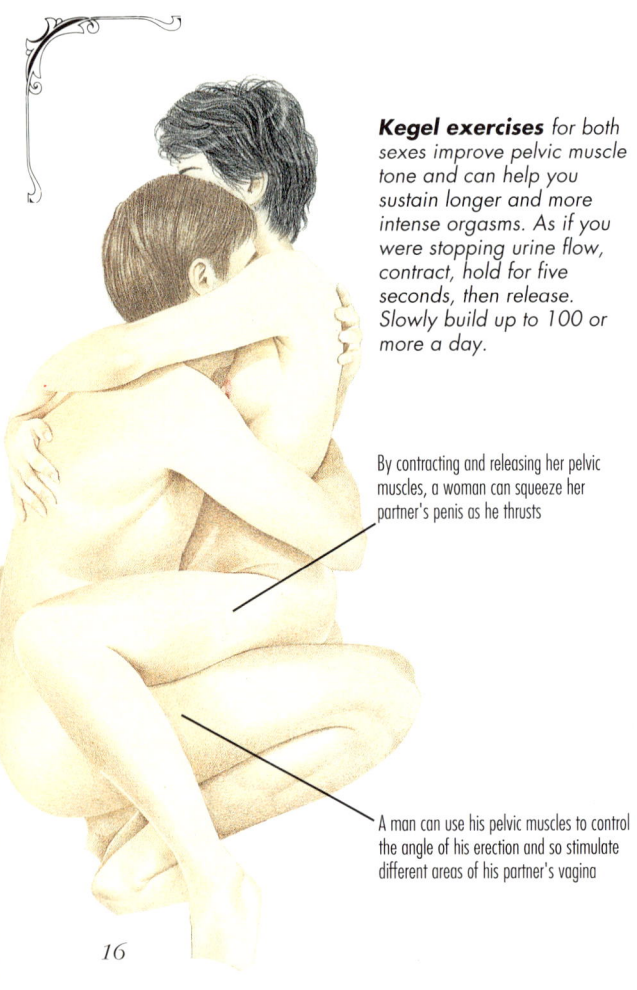

Kegel exercises for both sexes improve pelvic muscle tone and can help you sustain longer and more intense orgasms. As if you were stopping urine flow, contract, hold for five seconds, then release. Slowly build up to 100 or more a day.

By contracting and releasing her pelvic muscles, a woman can squeeze her partner's penis as he thrusts

A man can use his pelvic muscles to control the angle of his erection and so stimulate different areas of his partner's vagina

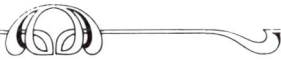

chapter two

SETTING THE SCENE

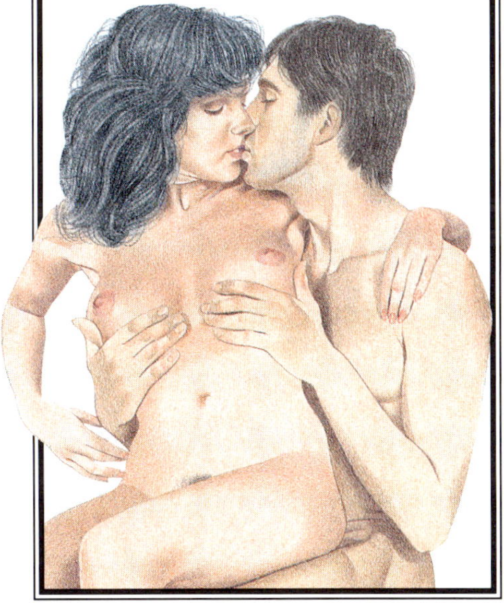

BATHING AND SHOWERING

From soaping each other in the shower to having slippery sex in a candle-lit bath, getting clean has never been so sensual.

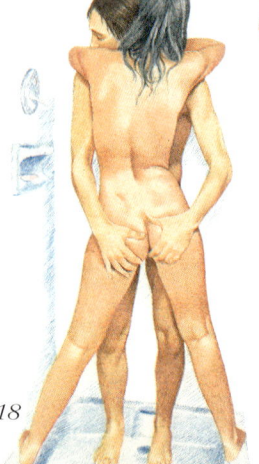

The buoyancy of water can make it easier to sustain more ambitious lovemaking positions in the bath by reducing the stress on joints and muscles.

Sex in the shower is very envigorating, but takes a lot of strength and control. Start by gently shampooing each other's hair, then let your hands wander.

Make love after bathing or showering while both of you are still wet and slippery and the room is still steamy.

Use the available furniture to support you as you thrust

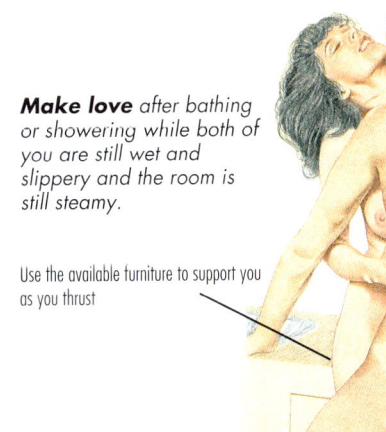

Enjoy the eroticism of food on your bodies – what you don't lick off you can wash off. Slowly melting ice cubes can trigger wonderful shivers of delight.

MASSAGE

Massage is a wonderful prelude to and extension of lovemaking. All areas of the body respond to its seductive effects.

In a warm, quiet room, explore, excite and sensuously relax your partner with varied strokes and touches. Experiment with different sensual textures – slip your hands into fake fur or rubber gloves, or caress your partner's skin with feathers or silk or velvet scarves, even a loofa. Smooth the skin with talcum powder for dry delicate softness or use scented oils for a more slippery sensation.

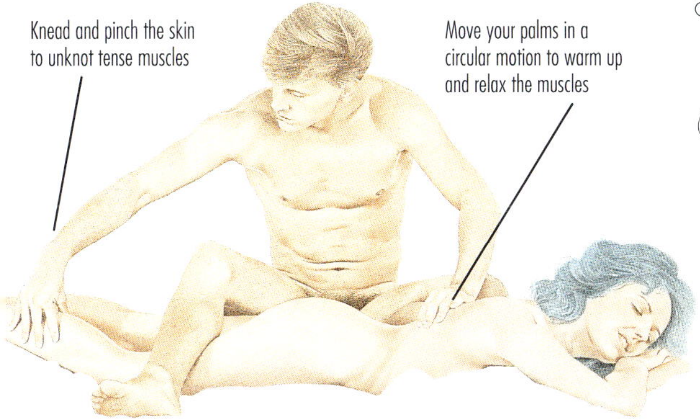

Knead and pinch the skin to unknot tense muscles

Move your palms in a circular motion to warm up and relax the muscles

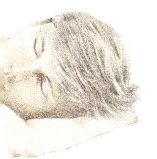

Tease your partner *into a state of arousal by deliberately avoiding the genitals when you give a massage. Beginning at the toes, slowly work your fingers in a gentle but firm circular motion along your partner's instep, ankle, calf, back of knee and up to the inner thigh. Keeping your fingers in contact with the body, switch your attention to the top of the body and work downwards, over the shoulders and arms, stomach and back.*

LOCATION

Sex is not just for the bedroom. Varying the location and time of day of your lovemaking can add excitement and adventure.

A cozy night in, set aside for a slow seduction in front of the fire, is a very romantic way to express your love, especially during the cold winter months. Set the scene by turning the lights down low and the heating up high.

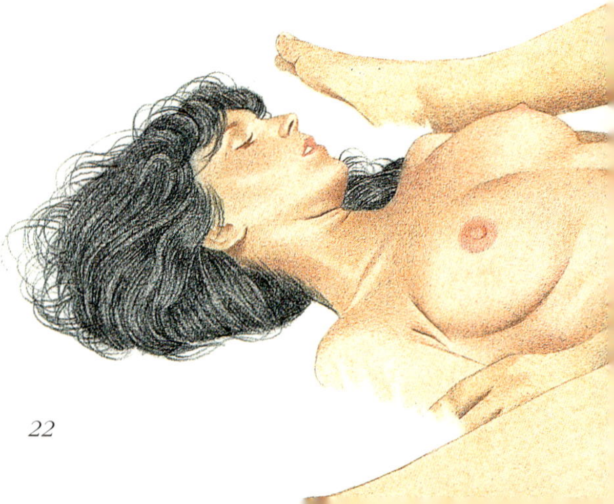

A warm room will help you to relax

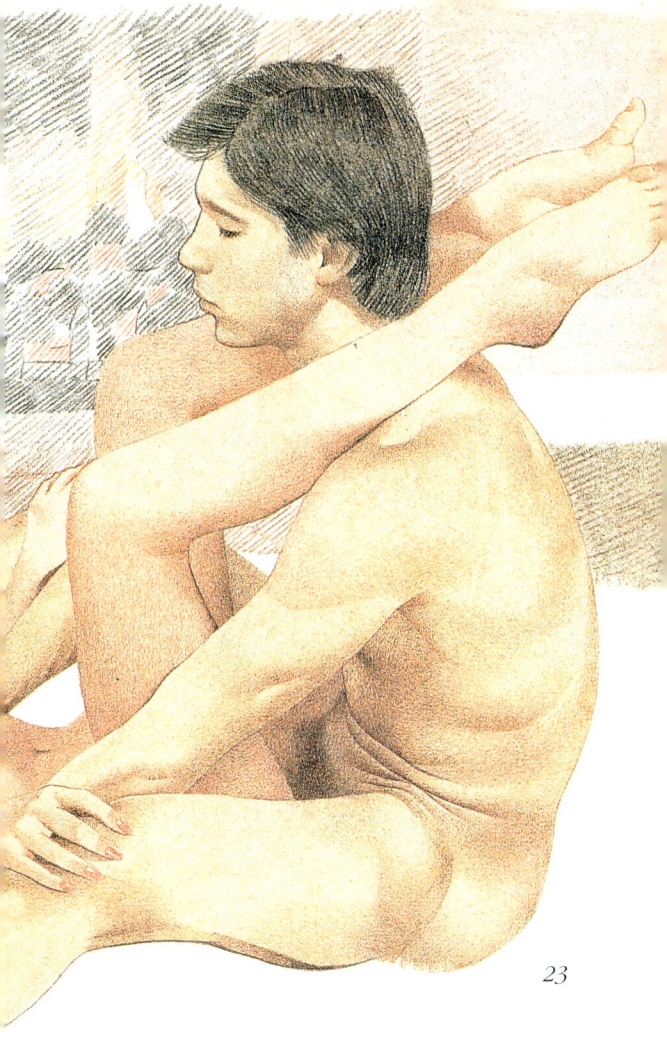

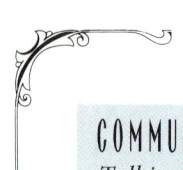

COMMUNICATION

Talking openly and honestly with your partner about your desires and feelings will help you achieve a more fulfilling love life.

Use eye contact to judge your partner's reactions

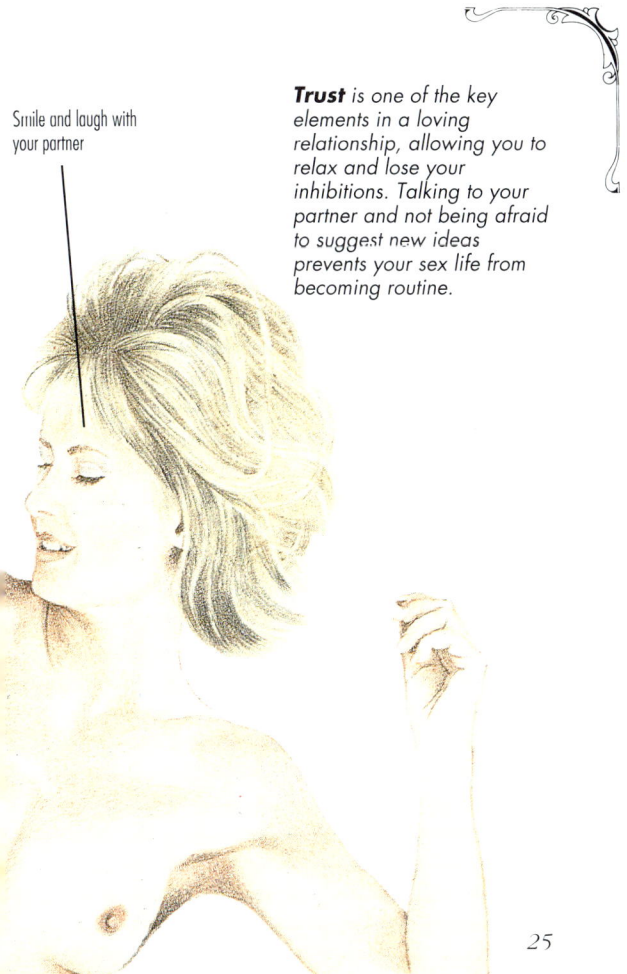

Smile and laugh with your partner

Trust is one of the key elements in a loving relationship, allowing you to relax and lose your inhibitions. Talking to your partner and not being afraid to suggest new ideas prevents your sex life from becoming routine.

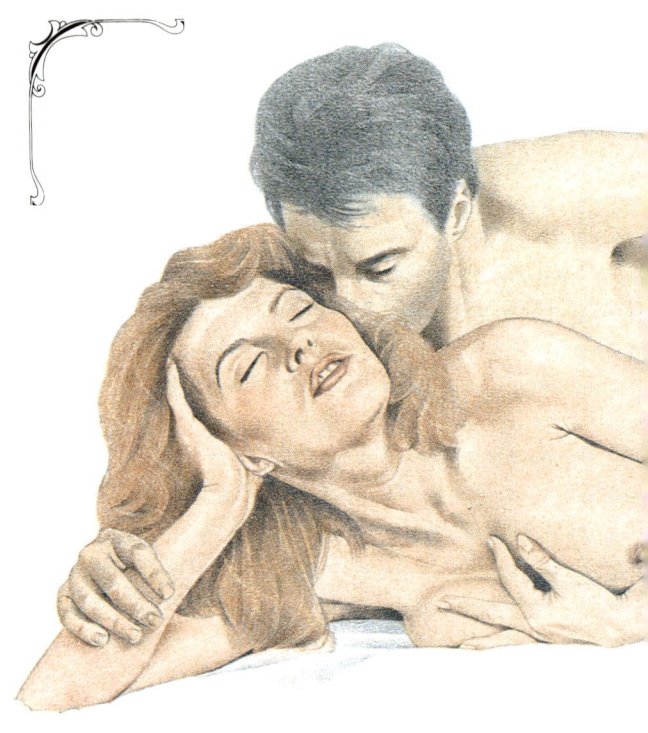

Non-verbal expression, *such as using and understanding body language, is also important – guiding your partner's hands is as effective as words. A discreet caress in a restaurant or a lingering glance at a party creates arousing sexual tension which can be brought to fulfillment later at home.*

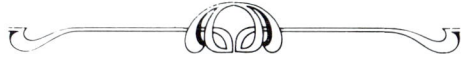

chapter three

FOREPLAY

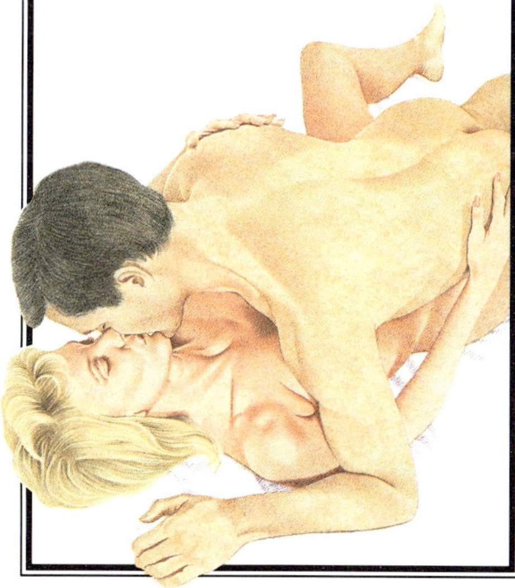

KISSING

Kissing is not only a demonstration of your love for your partner, but is a fundamental part of sexual arousal.

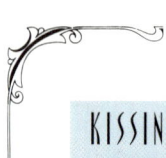

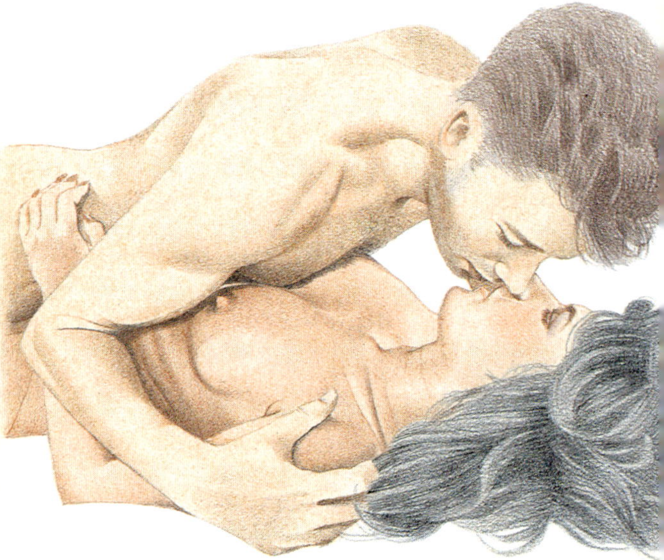

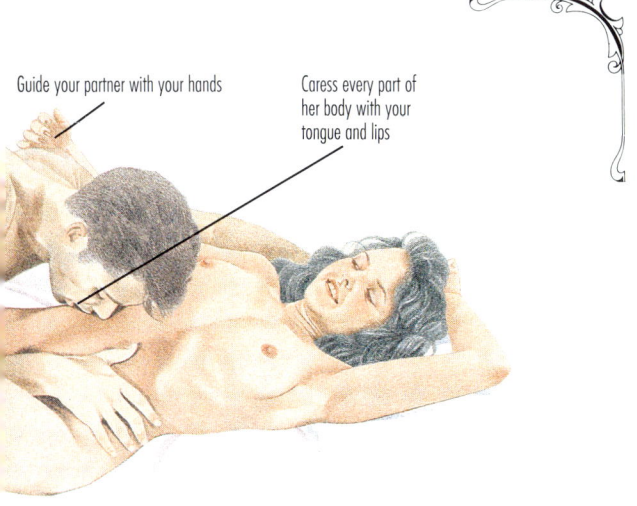

Guide your partner with your hands

Caress every part of her body with your tongue and lips

The lips, tongue, gums and inner mouth are all powerful erogenous zones. Mouth-to-mouth kisses can vary from teasing feather touches to possessively passionate or slow and searching ones. Deep, thrusting kisses can be as erotic as sex itself. French kissing is often neglected by couples who have been together a long time, but it is an excellent way of communicating your desire.

Body kisses are sex for the skin. Try maintaining body-mouth contact all during lovemaking, covering every inch of your partner's body with tender pecking kisses or slow, licking ones. Concentrate on less overtly sexual areas, such as the sides of the body and backs of the knees, as well as the more obvious breasts and genitals.

TOUCHING

Touching and being touched is an essential, delightfully sensual part of lovemaking. Caressing every inch of your partner's skin is erotically rewarding.

The fingertips contain a large number of nerve endings and are extremely sensitive. Use them to explore your partner's body and discover new erogenous zones. Let your partner guide you as to the places and kind of strokes that are the most pleasurable.

Touching is not just limited to the fingers. Caress, rub and tickle your partner with your lips, genitals, hair and feet. A woman can tease her partner by letting her breasts dangle over his body so that they lightly skim the surface of his skin.

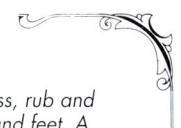

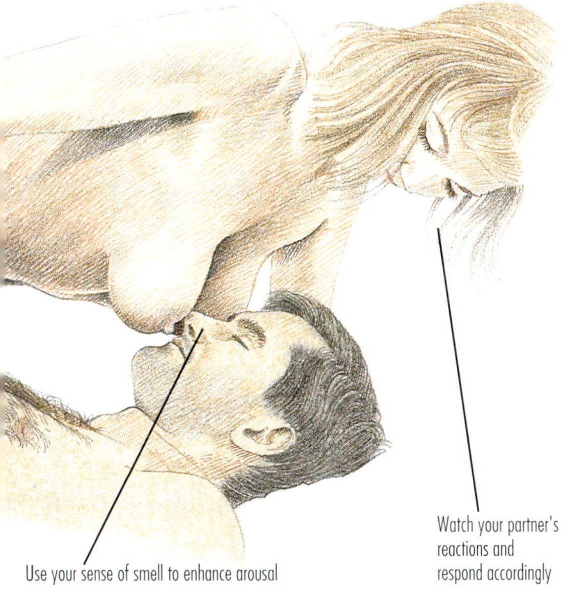

Use your sense of smell to enhance arousal

Watch your partner's reactions and respond accordingly

TONGUING

The tongue is a highly sensitive organ. It not only lets you feel and arouse your partner, but also enables you to taste them.

Deliberately, slowly, move over every part of your partner's body with long, catlike licks, from forehead down to toes on each side, then back up the front of the body. Finish with extra attention at the genitals to bring them to a full state of arousal.

Skin-to-skin contact increases sexual arousal

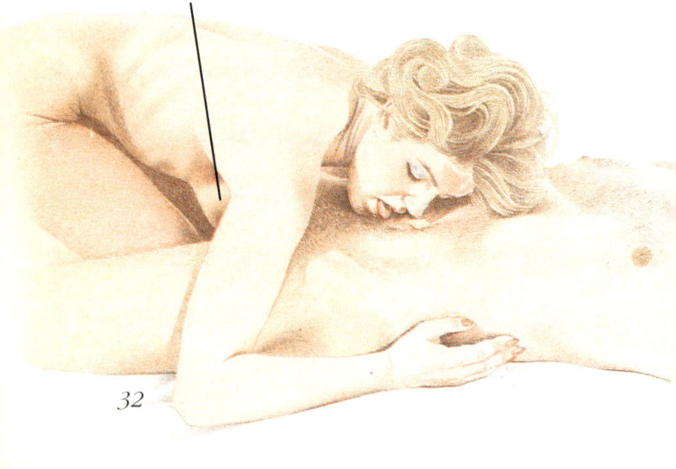

The soft skin of the inner thigh, as well as the inner arm, crease of the elbow, wrists and backs of the knees (indeed, anywhere the pulse is tangible), is particularly responsive to your tongue work.

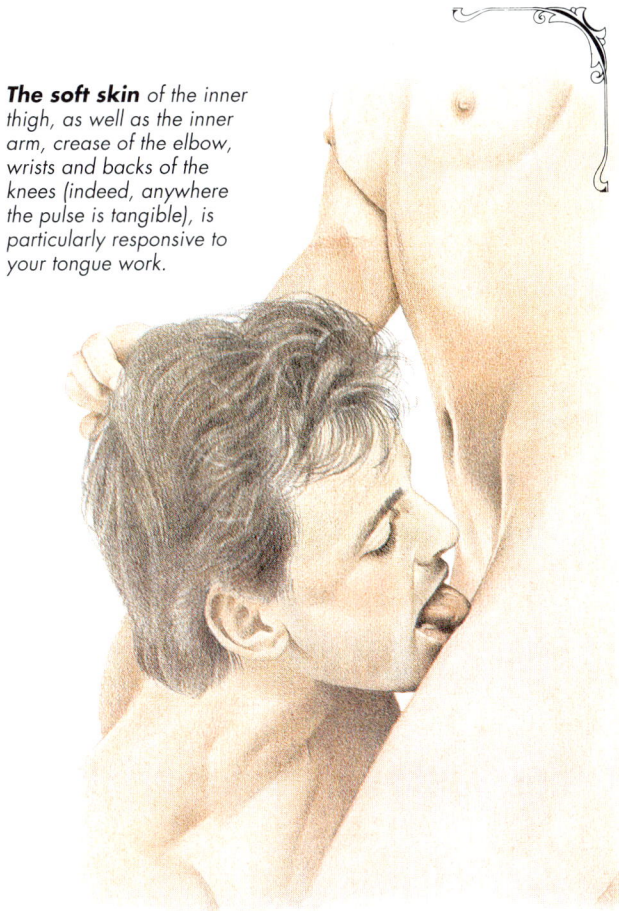

UNDRESSING

Add an erotic, teasing touch to your lovemaking by suggestively disrobing in front of your partner. Alternatively, opt to be undressed by them.

Take it in turns to undress and be undressed, enjoying the switch from being passive to active. As you undress yourself, increase eroticism by first looking away and pretending your partner is not there, then openly flaunting your nakedness. Experiment with exotic lingerie, flickering candlelight and sexy music.

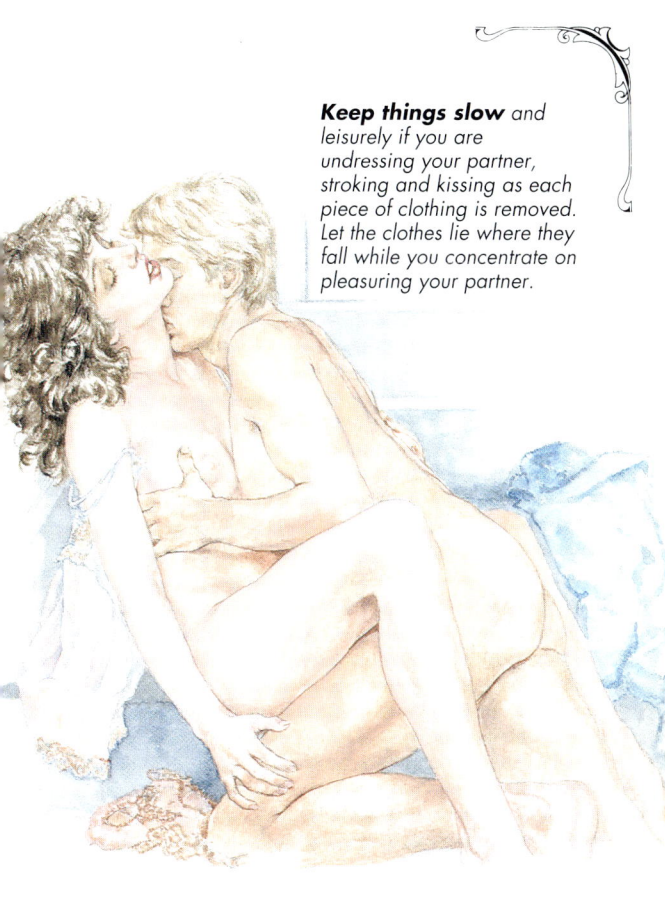

Keep things slow and leisurely if you are undressing your partner, stroking and kissing as each piece of clothing is removed. Let the clothes lie where they fall while you concentrate on pleasuring your partner.

MASTURBATION

Masturbation is not only pleasurable, it is one of the best ways to explore your sexual responses. Share your preferences for greater mutual enjoyment.

Discover the erotic potential of your body by examining your genitalia with your eyes as well as your hands. Women can use a mirror to help them gain a better view.

Female masturbation
Whether by brushing the clitoris with a fingertip or by massaging the whole area with the hand, most women will be able to bring themselves to orgasm.

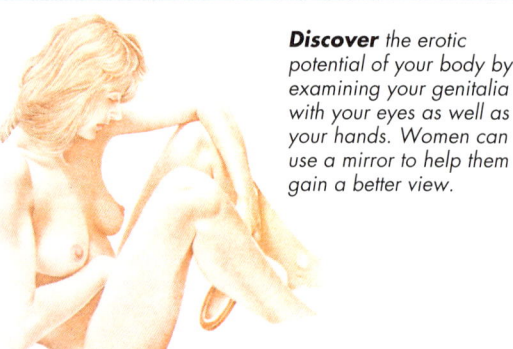

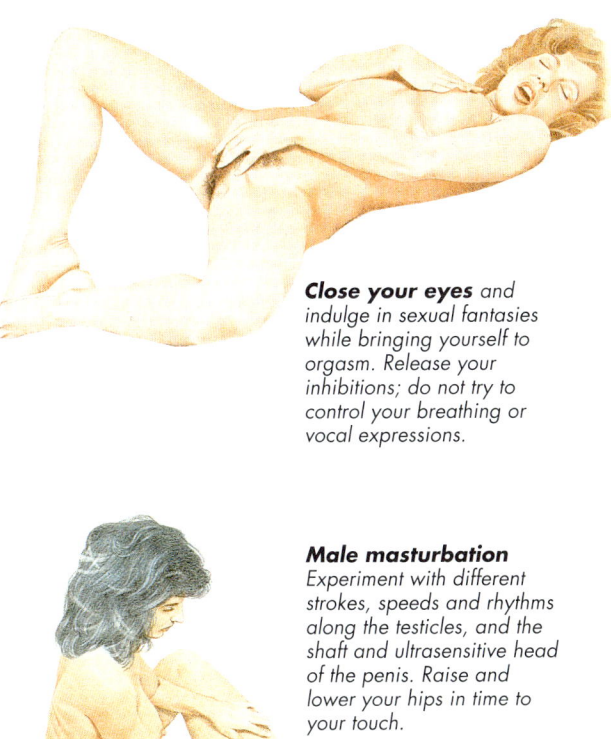

Close your eyes and indulge in sexual fantasies while bringing yourself to orgasm. Release your inhibitions; do not try to control your breathing or vocal expressions.

Male masturbation
Experiment with different strokes, speeds and rhythms along the testicles, and the shaft and ultrasensitive head of the penis. Raise and lower your hips in time to your touch.

Mutual masturbation (him to her)
Stroke your partner's vaginal entrance and labia before gently massaging her clitoris. Slightly increase the tempo and pressure as she approaches orgasm. Let her guide your hand with hers.

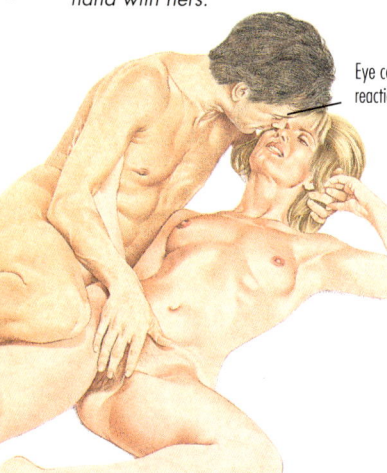

Eye contact is necessary to judge her reactions

Caress her whole body,
stimulating other erogenous zones such as the breasts and nipples, for more intense sensations. By sitting behind your partner you can mimic her favorite touches more easily.

Mutual masturbation (her to him)

Caress your partner's testes and anal area, then massage the shaft of his penis with firm, rhythmic movements. Stimulate the head and frenulum as his arousal increases.

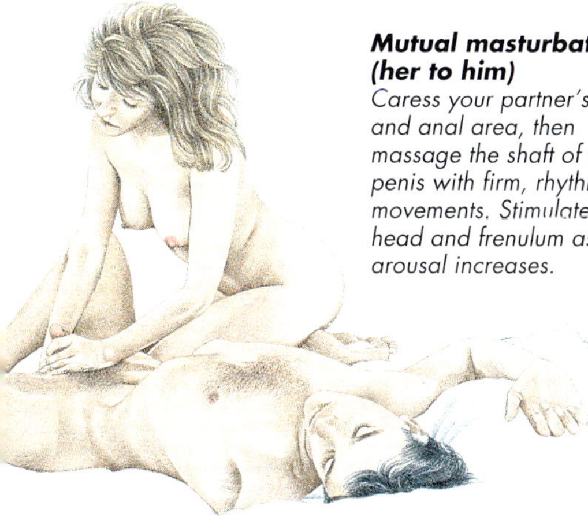

Take things slowly:
use oils, luxuriate in the sensation; fantasize.

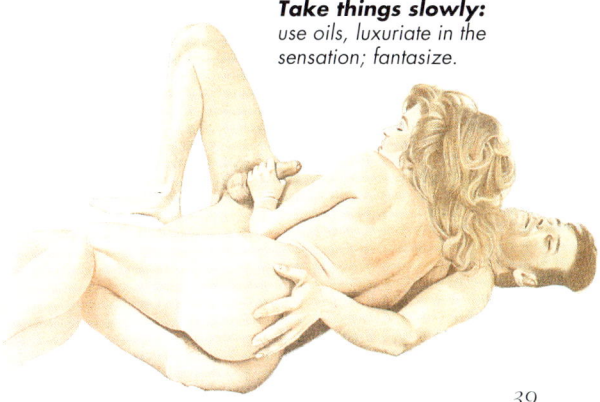

Masturbating each other to a climax is a wonderfully satisfying part of – or alternative to – intercourse. It is 'safe sex' and, because you can more easily manipulate each other's responses, you can learn what most effectively arouses your partner for the most stimulating reaction. Be imaginative: try using a vibrator or the spray from the showerhead as an aid to arousal.

Use a firm, pumping action on his penis

Open yourself up to your partner physically and emotionally

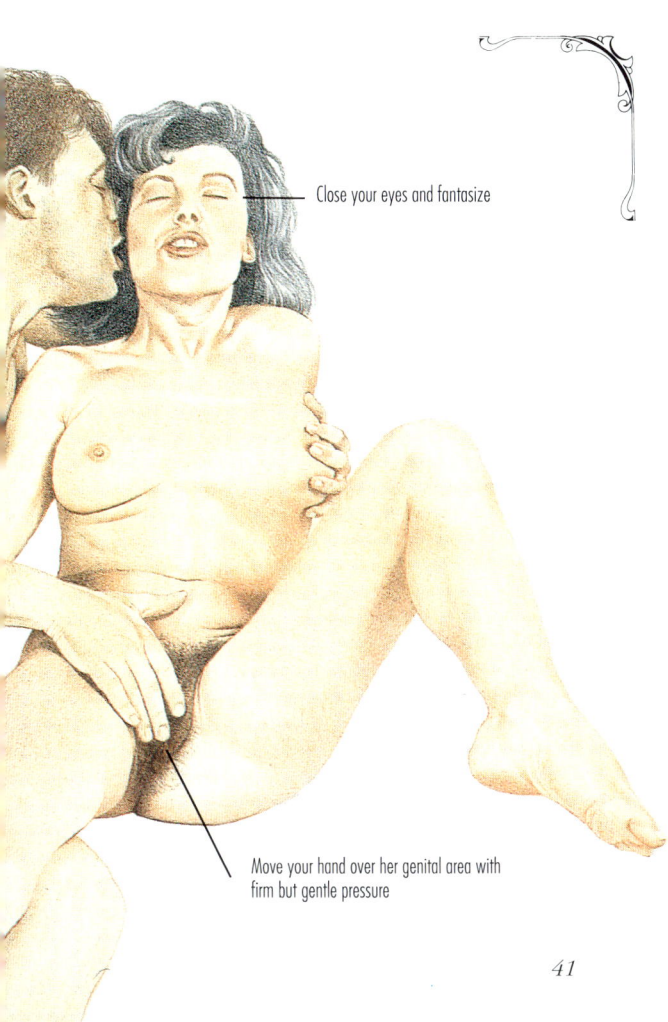

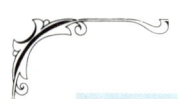

EROGENOUS ZONES

The biggest erogenous zone is your imagination. But every inch of your body can be licked, caressed or rubbed to stimulate the erotic senses.

Many areas of the body that are responsive to erotic stimulation – mouth and lips, ears, breasts and genitals, for example – are shared by most people, while others can be distinctive, even unusual, involving areas that are not conventionally sexual. Discover them languorously, sensuously, on your own or with your partner.

For many women, stimulation of erogenous zones other than the genitals can be enough to bring them to orgasm, and some can climax through fantasy alone. For most men, although sexual activity is centred much more on the genital region, stimulation of other sensitive areas can help increase arousal.

Make sex
a whole-body experience. A woman's breasts can form a sensuous channel for her partner's penis. In this position, his pubic hairs can simultaneously tickle her nipples into a state of arousal.

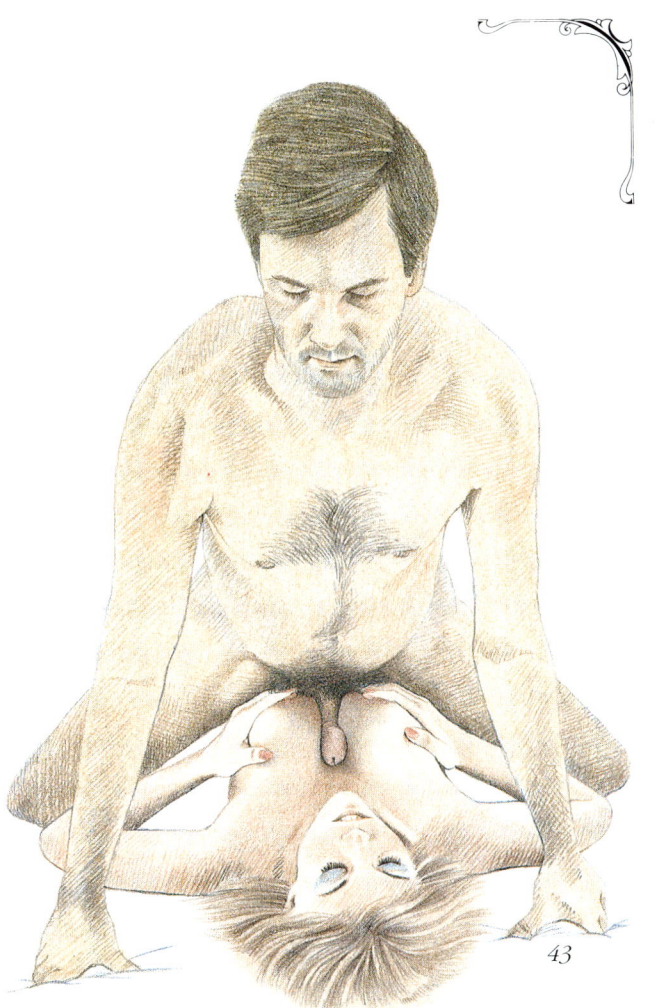

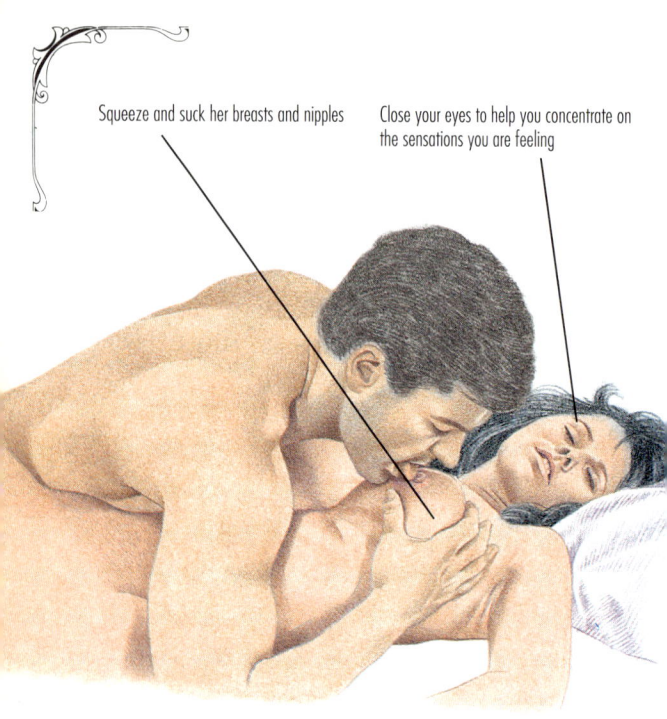

Squeeze and suck her breasts and nipples

Close your eyes to help you concentrate on the sensations you are feeling

Breasts and nipples *are one of the major erogenous zones for both men and women. Most women like to have them stimulated during lovemaking, as the nipple, aureole and whole breast area are extremely sensitive to touch. Squeezing, kissing, licking, even blowing, can be extremely arousing and sensual.*

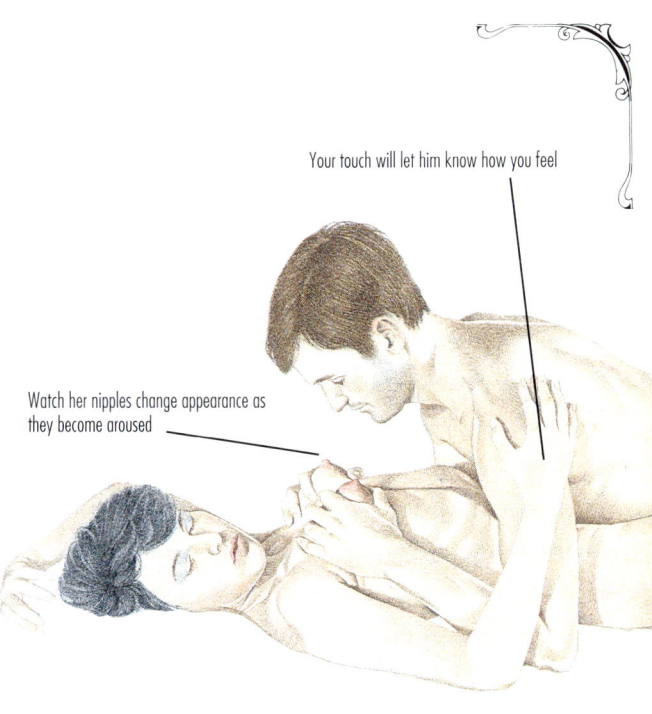

Your touch will let him know how you feel

Watch her nipples change appearance as they become aroused

The nipples become erect and harden when they are stimulated, as blood gorges the tissues. Their colour also darkens. Some women like to have their breasts firmly handled and squeezed, while others prefer a gentler, stroking touch. Let your partner guide you as to the kind of touch that she finds most enjoyable.

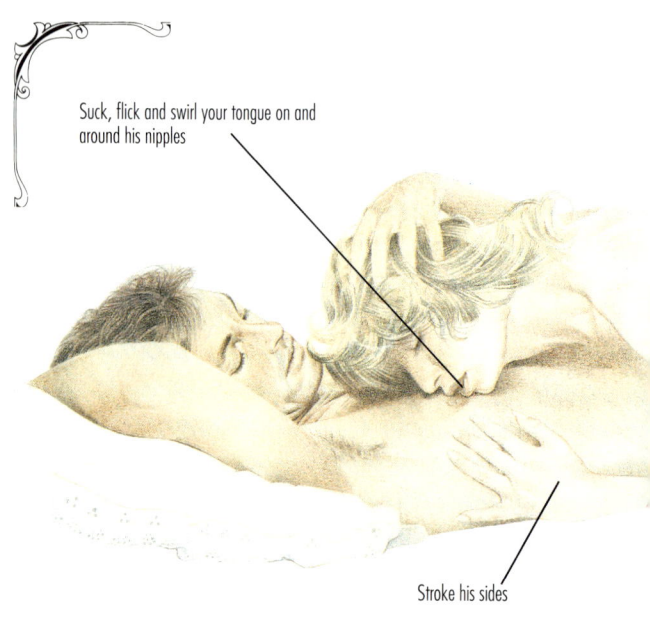

Suck, flick and swirl your tongue on and around his nipples

Stroke his sides

A man's chest, especially his nipples, can be responsive to stroking and kissing. Moisten his nipples with your saliva or perhaps some wine, and tease them with your tongue while you caress his chest.
Alternatively, caress your partner's nipples with your own breasts or rub them with your labia.

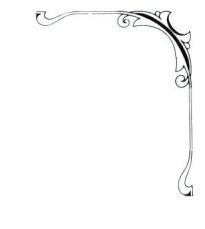

The soft inner thighs
are extremely sensitive to stimulation. Run the length of them with your tongue, giving feathery kisses. Suck, lick and tease the backs of the knees, then move back up to the genitals, lightly brushing the pubic hairs, and work back down.

Nuzzle against her genitals as you suck and lick her inner thighs

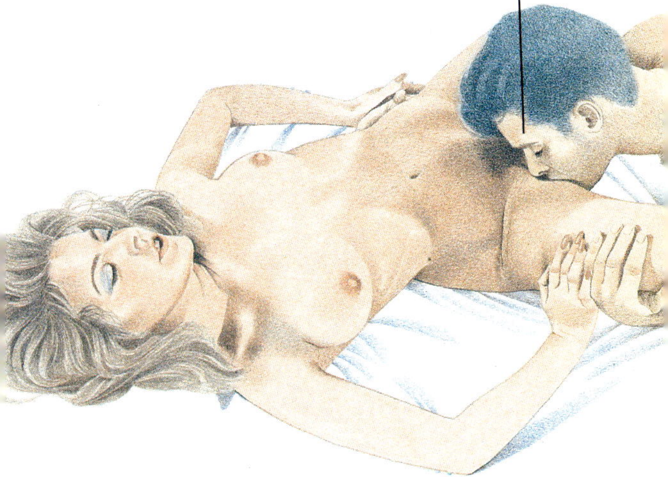

Feet and toes can respond pleasurably to kissing, rubbing and sucking. Some people find their feet too sensitive to enjoy attention there, while others find it immensely arousing. Keep strokes positive and strong to avoid tickling your partner. Toes are erogenic – perfect for sensuous licking and sucking – particularly the areas between them.

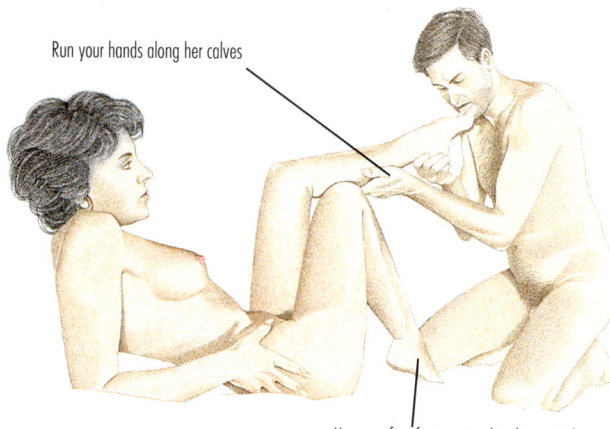

Run your hands along her calves

Use your free foot to stimulate his genitals

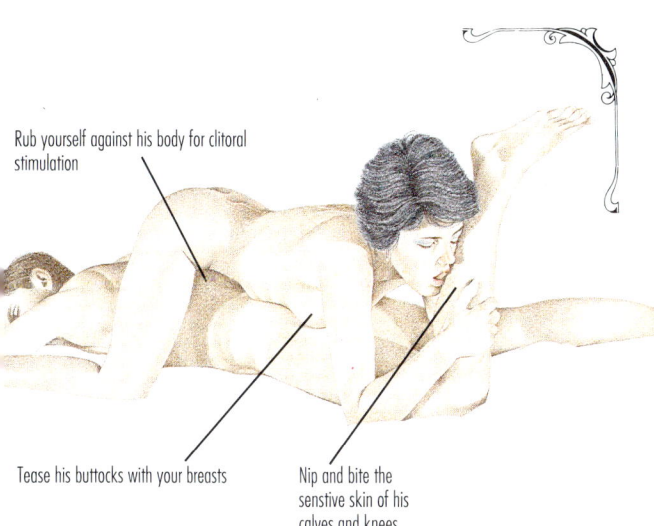

Rub yourself against his body for clitoral stimulation

Tease his buttocks with your breasts

Nip and bite the sensitive skin of his calves and knees

The back of the body contains fewer nerve endings than the front, but is still responsive to touch. The head and neck area is especially sensitive; use soft, feathery strokes with the lips, tongue and fingertips across the nape, sides and back of the neck, not forgetting the ear lobes. Progress to firmer, nipping caresses across the shoulders and down the back, sides, buttocks, anus and legs.

The small of the back is surprisingly sensitive for many people, and will respond pleasurably to being flicked and brushed with the hair. Gentle to firm scratching down the length of the back can be very arousing to both sexes.

The skin is our biggest sexual organ, so it is important to try to maintain as much body-to-body contact as you can while making love. The skin is exquisitely responsive to a great variety of textures and temperatures. Drizzle warm honey or cold wine on your partner's body; caress it with slippery satin, rough body brushes, soft feathers, smooth rubber – they all arouse the responses and awaken the nerve-endings.

Employ all your senses to discover your partner and increase your excitement. Smell the muskiness under the arms or around the genitals; taste the saltiness of the labia and the cheesiness of the feet. Let your body relax and respond instinctively.

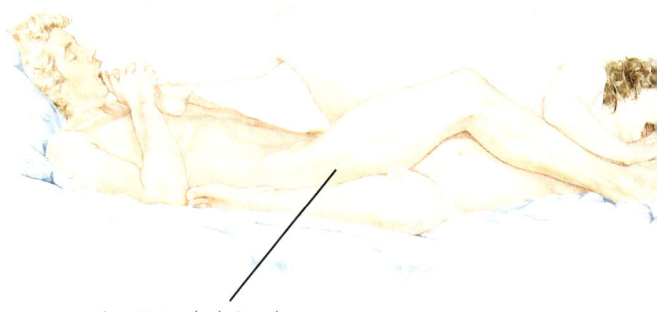

Luxuriate in each other's touch

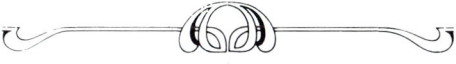

chapter four

POSITIONS & PERFORMANCE

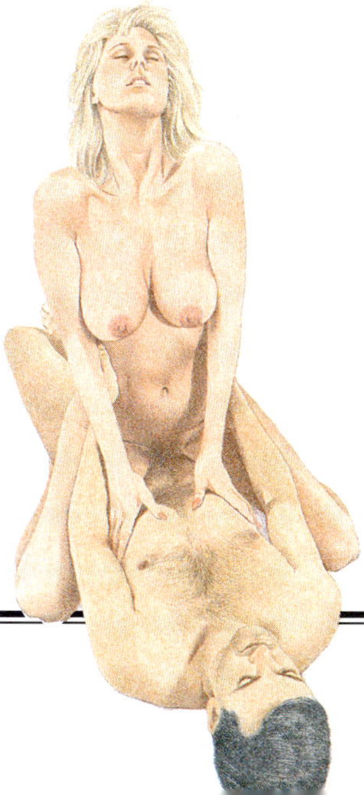

ORAL SEX

Oral sex is especially intimate, as well as erotically satisfying. The tongue, lips and mouth are gentler, and can be more flexible, on the genitals than the fingers.

Fellatio Performed by women on men. Using your saliva as lubricant and taking care not to bite, stimulate your partner's penis by sucking, licking and rhythmically 'pumping' it with your mouth. Run your tongue along the shaft, especially around the head and frenulum. Increase your speed as he becomes more aroused. Switch to manual stimulation or intercourse at this point, if your partner is not wearing a condom and you do not want him to ejaculate in your mouth.

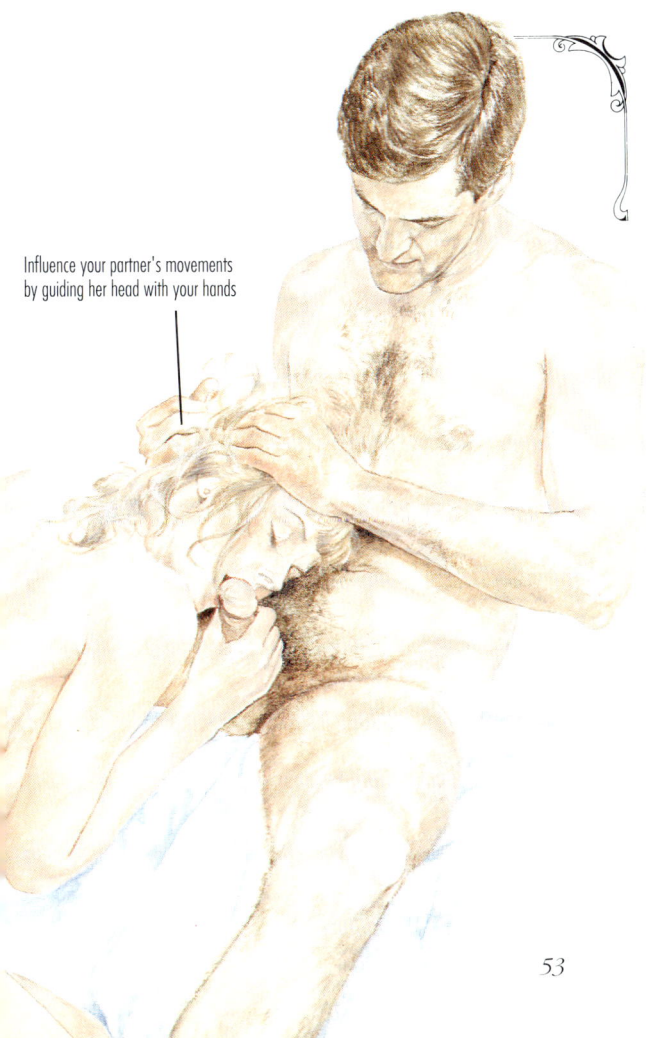

Influence your partner's movements by guiding her head with your hands

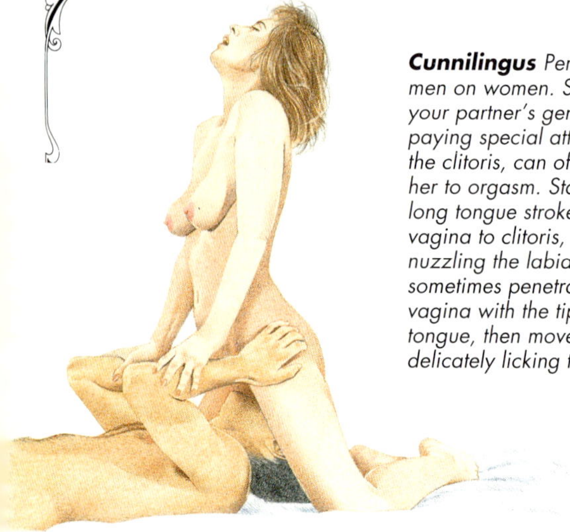

Cunnilingus Performed by men on women. Stimulating your partner's genital area, paying special attention to the clitoris, can often arouse her to orgasm. Start with long tongue strokes from the vagina to clitoris, gently nuzzling the labia and sometimes penetrating the vagina with the tip of your tongue, then move on to delicately licking the clitoris.

Be guided by your partner. Respond to her sounds and movements.

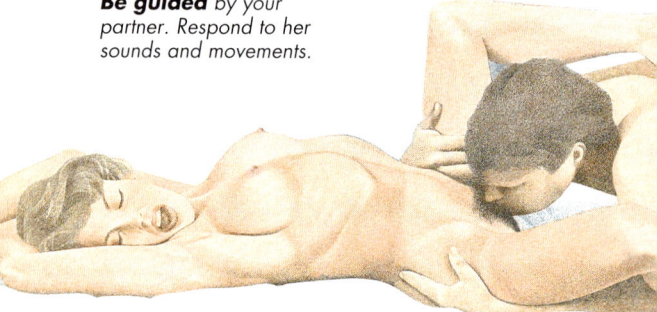

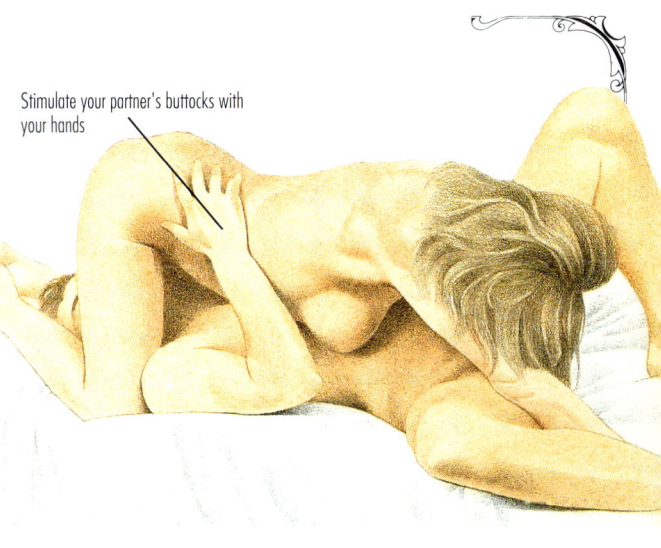

Stimulate your partner's buttocks with your hands

'Soixante-neuf' or '69' Partner-to-partner genital mouth work needs some restraint, or one of you could get carried away and be bitten or hurt. As with aiming for simultaneous orgasm, some couples enjoy the mutual mounting excitement, while others find it more sexually exciting to focus upon one partner's pleasure at a time.

Vary your position according to mood, so that sometimes the man, sometimes the woman is on top. Alternatively, both partners can lie side-by-side.

WOMAN DOMINANT

Being on top allows the woman to take a more active role in lovemaking. She can control the type and speed of movement and depth of penetration.

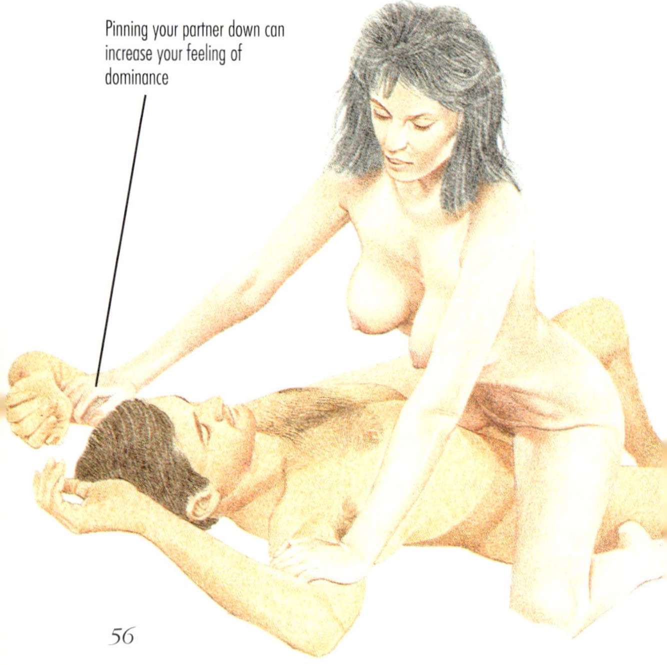

Pinning your partner down can increase your feeling of dominance

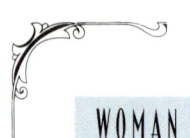

Facing away By having her back to her partner, as she sits astride him, knees up, the woman can regulate the depth of his thrusts, and can also massage her clitoris for extra arousal. Although the position is not considered an intimate one, with faces turned away, it allows for better fantasizing. He has a full, appreciative view of her bottom, and can caress her back and sides.

Use your hands to lift yourself up and to massage your clitoris and your partner's scrotum

Reverse missionary
By sitting atop her partner and facing him, the woman can move up and down to raise and lower herself on his penis. Backward and forward movement will stimulate her vaginal walls and clitoris.

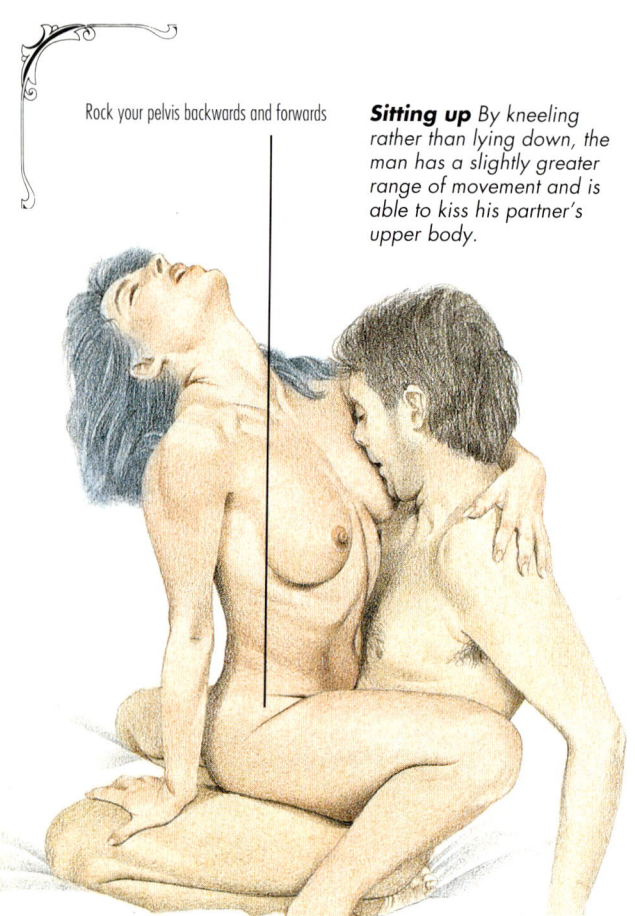

Rock your pelvis backwards and forwards

Sitting up By kneeling rather than lying down, the man has a slightly greater range of movement and is able to kiss his partner's upper body.

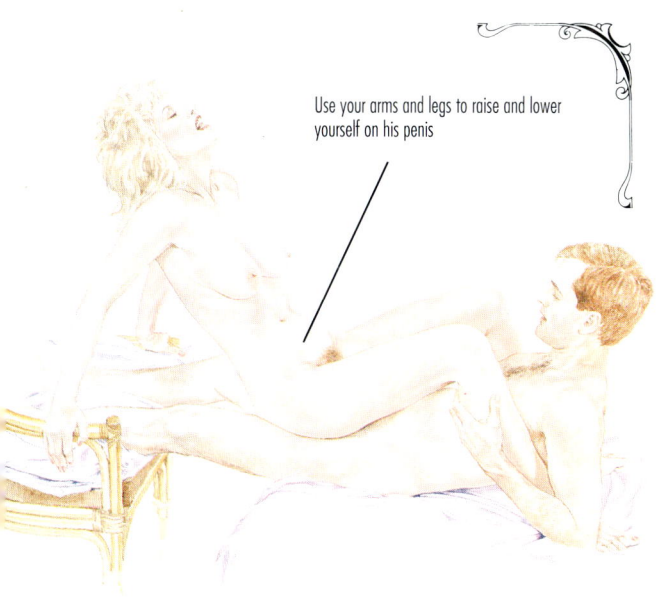

Use your arms and legs to raise and lower yourself on his penis

'Scissors' Facing her partner and half-sitting, half-lying backwards, insures not only a good angle for stimulation to both partners, but also visual stimulation to him, as he can more easily see her genital area and his penis sliding in and out as he thrusts upward and she downward. He can massage her clitoris with his hand, and she has good leverage to control the kind of stimulation she wants for a satisfying orgasm.

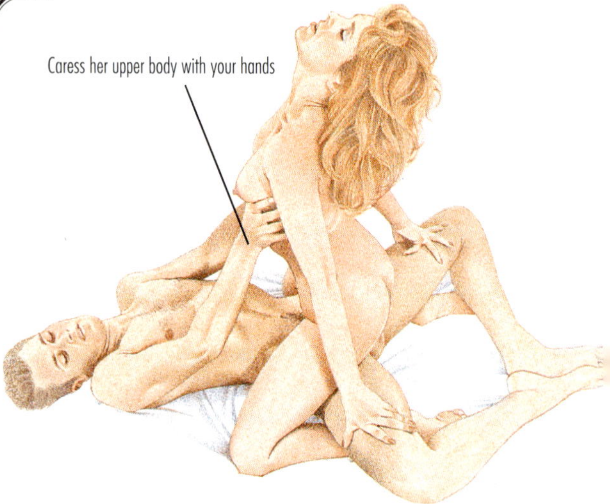

Caress her upper body with your hands

On knees If she takes some of the weight on her knees, placed on either side of her partner's hips, the woman is free to create more stimulation for her pubic area. By sitting up, she can vary the angle of penetration, and so adjust the feeling for each of them.

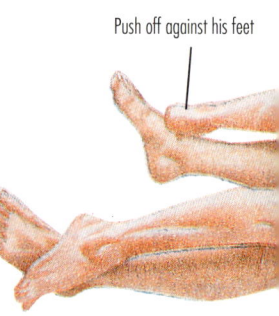

Push off against his feet

The 'frog' This position allows full contact along both partners' bodies. By resting her feet on her partner's and supporting herself on her hands, the woman can raise and lower herself to rub her clitoris against her partner's groin for stimulation. By lying in between his legs, she has less freedom of movement but can grip his penis tightly with her thighs and move enough for the shaft of the penis to stimulate her clitoris.

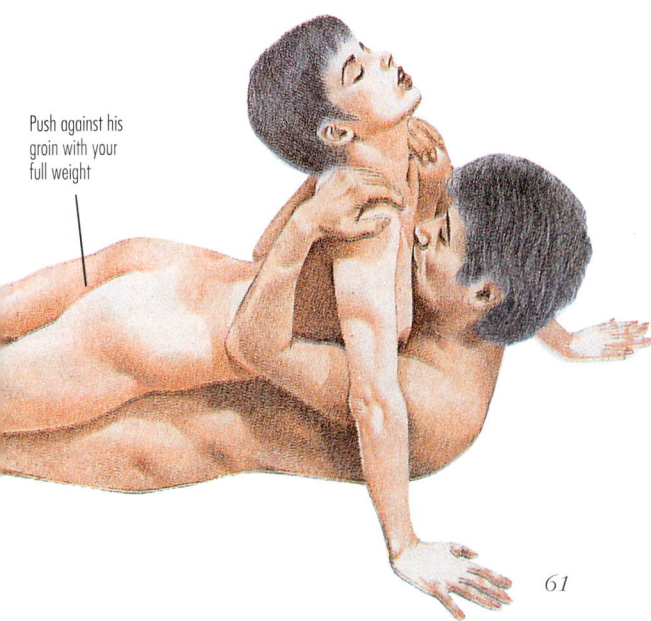

Push against his groin with your full weight

MAN DOMINANT

Man-on-top positions are popular because they allow the man flexibility while staying inside his partner. Penetration is also variable: deep or shallow, rough or gentle.

Missionary position As he lies on top of his partner, between her thighs, the man takes the more active role in lovemaking, since he has more control of his movements. He should take some weight on his elbows or arms, to allow her more comfort. By clenching her buttocks and thrusting upwards while simultaneously swivelling her hips, the woman may be able to orgasm more quickly. If pillows are used to support her hips, the woman can tilt her pelvis upwards to make the vagina more accessible and so allow slightly deeper penetration.

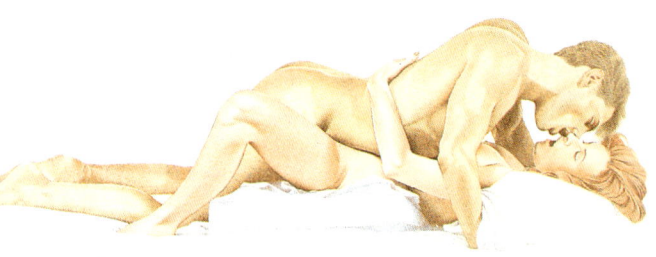

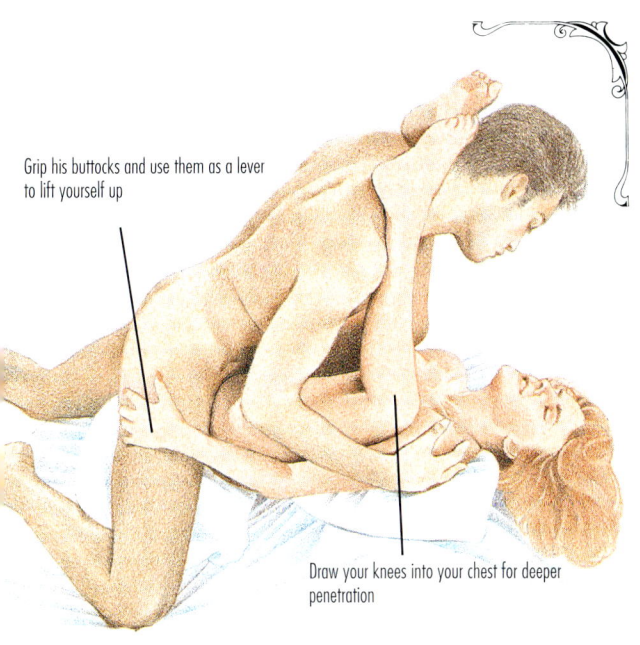

Grip his buttocks and use them as a lever to lift yourself up

Draw your knees into your chest for deeper penetration

Feet on shoulders As she wraps her legs around his neck, the woman's pelvis is tilted upwards, enabling deeper penetration. She should be sufficiently stimulated so that her vagina is fully opened, otherwise her partner's thrusting could be uncomfortable. If he leans forward, his pubic bone can rub against her for more erotic stimulation. With such deep penetration, the man's semen is deposited right at the opening of the cervix when he ejaculates, making this a good position for couples who want to conceive.

'Parting of the waves' Although movement by both partners is limited, this position allows a unique angle of penetration, with the penis stimulating the back wall of the vagina. To take up the position, the woman should lie back near the edge of the bed and raise her legs in the air. Her partner should kneel astride her, facing away, then lean forward as he enters her, taking his weight on his hands on the floor. The woman can use her hands to caress her partner's thighs and buttocks and to stimulate his anus, as well as to assist his thrusting.

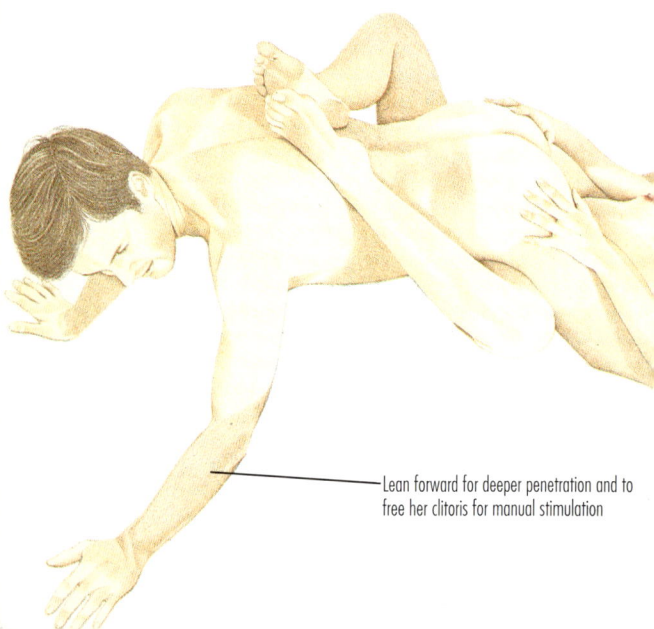

Lean forward for deeper penetration and to free her clitoris for manual stimulation

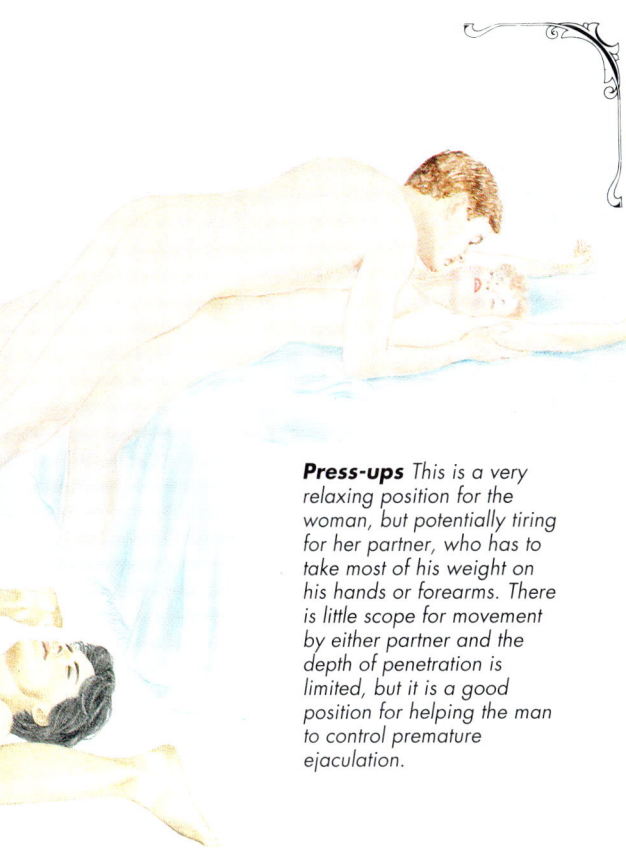

Press-ups This is a very relaxing position for the woman, but potentially tiring for her partner, who has to take most of his weight on his hands or forearms. There is little scope for movement by either partner and the depth of penetration is limited, but it is a good position for helping the man to control premature ejaculation.

'Crossed swords' This position allows the man to enter his partner at a slight angle, and so stimulate the side walls of her vagina. By leaning back and taking the weight on their hands, partners have a greater opportunity to move and to watch each other's reactions. The clitoris is exposed for extra stimulation, although upper body contact is almost impossible without restricting genital stimulation.

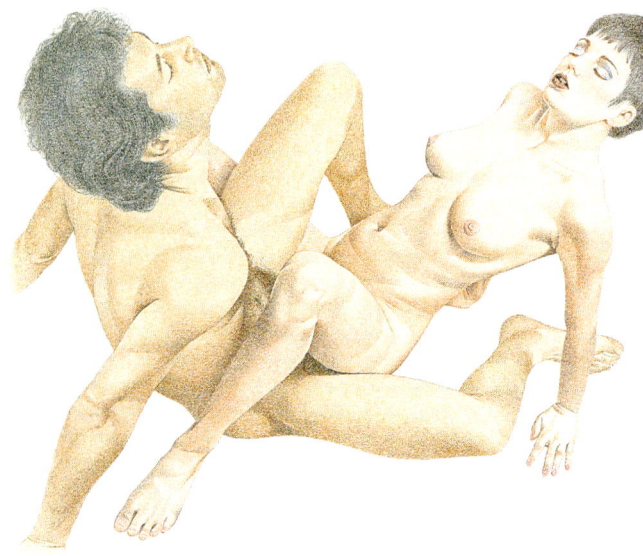

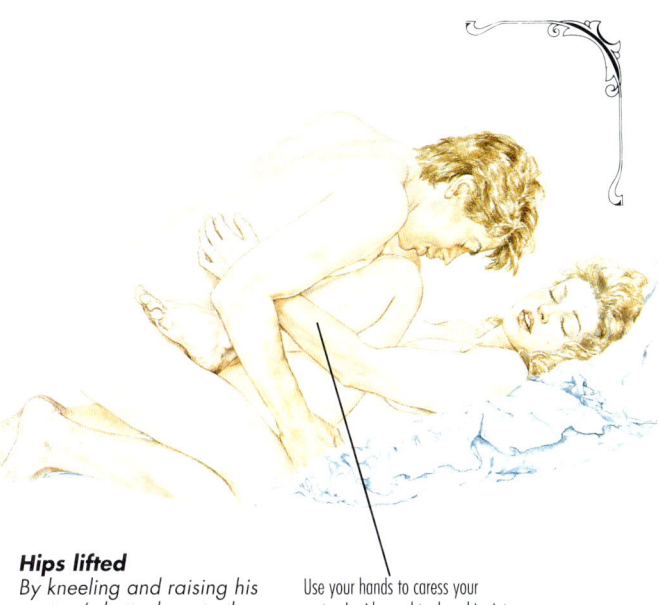

Hips lifted
By kneeling and raising his partner's buttocks onto the lower part of his thighs as he enters her, and then supporting her hips with both hands, the man can penetrate her in such a way as to stimulate the highly sensitive front wall of her vagina, where the G-spot is situated. The woman can deepen penetration by drawing her knees up into her chest.

Use your hands to caress your partner's sides and to draw him into you as he thrusts

REAR ENTRY

These positions enable deeper penetration and more intense stimulation of the front vaginal wall. Most allow good access to the clitoris for manual stimulation.

Lying flat (woman on top) By slowly and gently leaning back onto her partner, after first lowering herself onto his penis, the woman can receive added stimulation from his hands stroking her clitoris, stomach and breasts. The full-length skin contact is arousing, and many men enjoy the sensation of being dominated when pinned down by the weight of their partner. Penetration is not deep, but the penis does stimulate the sensitive front wall of the vagina quite intensely.

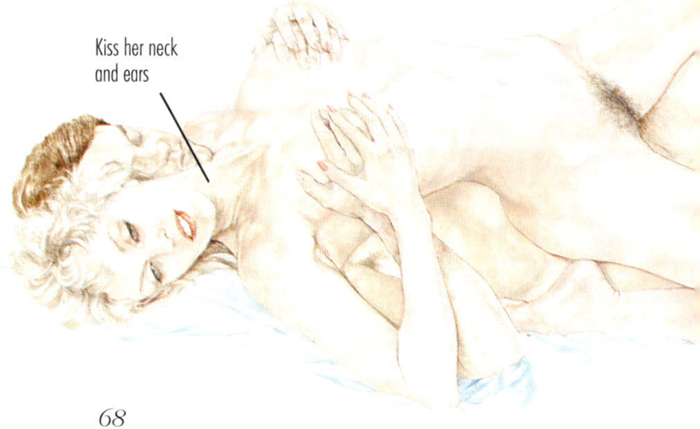

Kiss her neck and ears

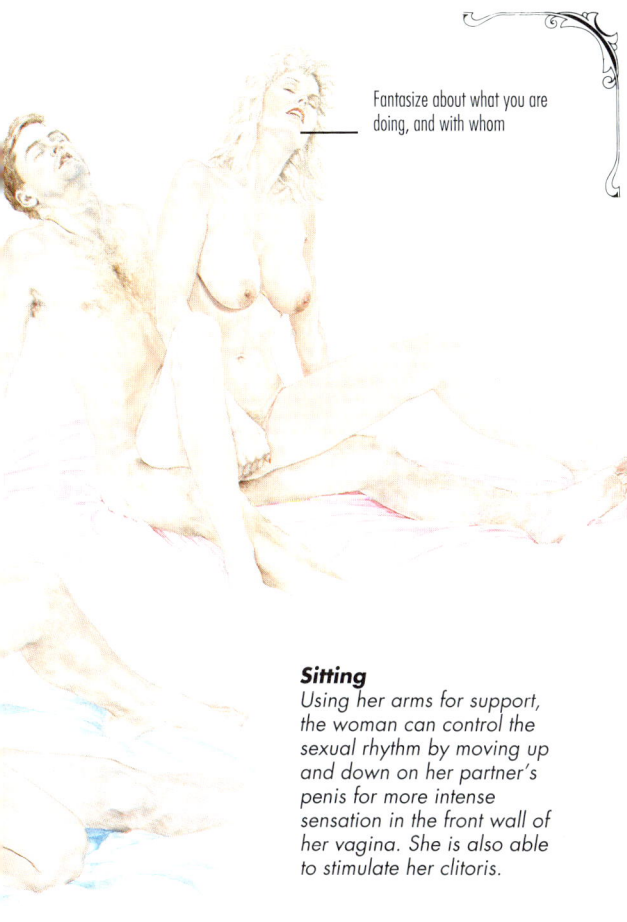

Fantasize about what you are doing, and with whom

Sitting
Using her arms for support, the woman can control the sexual rhythm by moving up and down on her partner's penis for more intense sensation in the front wall of her vagina. She is also able to stimulate her clitoris.

'Doggy' This position is one of the best for achieving maximum-depth penetration. It allows the man to thrust fully, and the woman can vary the sensation by how wide or narrow she opens her legs. Many women are excited by the sense of abandonment that they feel when being taken from behind, and indulge in fantasies of domination and anonymity. Care should be taken that it is not painful for the woman, and it is not recommended for women who have weak backs, or are in an advanced stage of pregnancy.

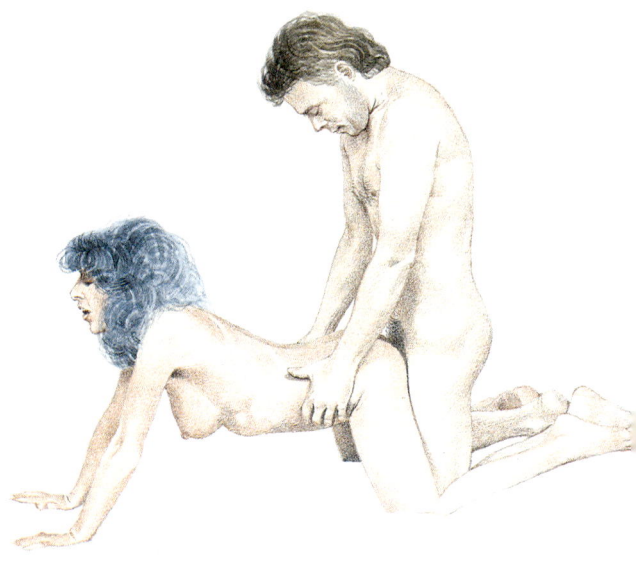

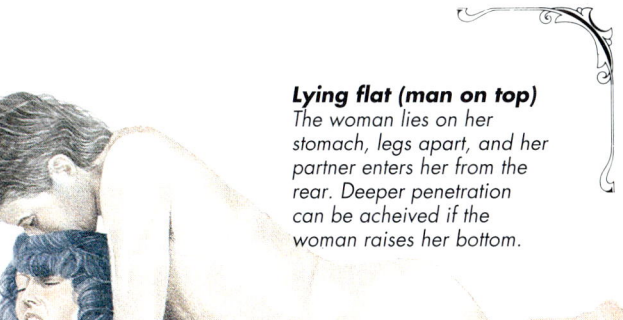

Lying flat (man on top)
The woman lies on her stomach, legs apart, and her partner enters her from the rear. Deeper penetration can be acheived if the woman raises her bottom.

Arch your and back and push backwards onto his penis

Use your full weight to thrust deeply

Upright 'doggy'
The woman leans against a bed or chair so that her partner can more easily fondle her breasts and stroke her body.

SIDE-BY-SIDE

While penetration is relatively shallow, side-by-side positions can make lovemaking more leisurely, for extra arousal. They also allow for intimate caressing.

Lying with legs raised This position allows for good visual stimulation to the man, and leaves both partners' hands free to caress each other. He can easily reach her breasts and clitoris, and can enjoy her expressions of affection and sexual excitement. Penetration is shallow, so the woman should hold her legs tightly closed to avoid letting his penis slip out.

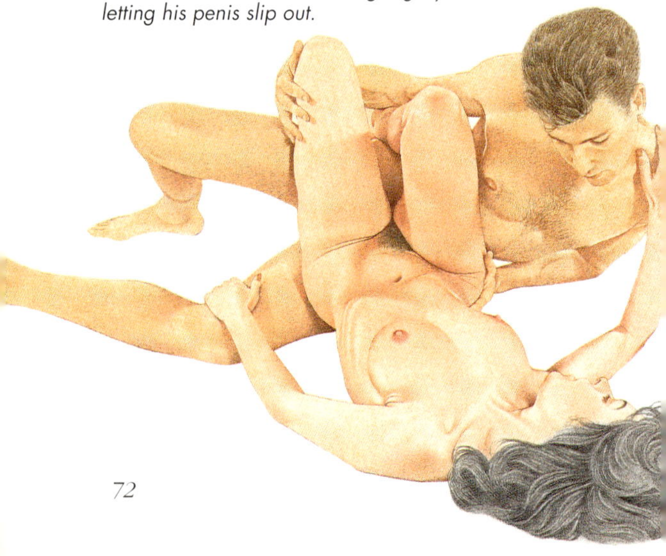

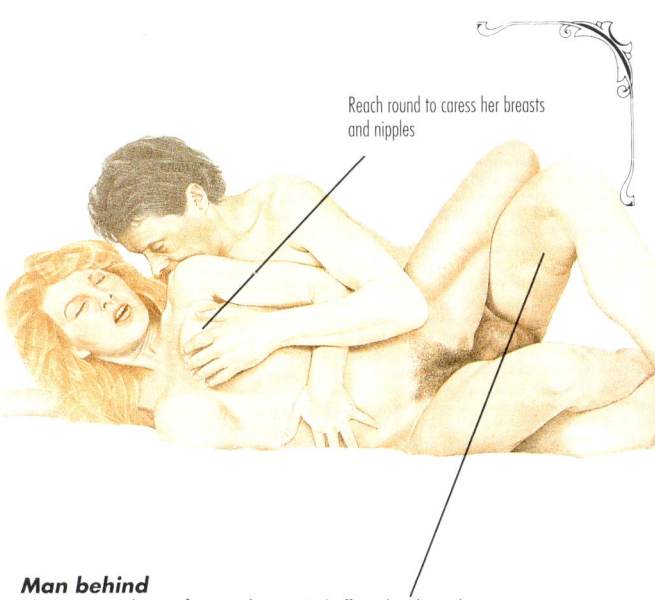

Reach round to caress her breasts and nipples

Push off your bent leg to thrust

Man behind
The woman leans forward on her hip to make penetration easier, and the man raises his outside leg to make it easier for him to thrust. By drawing her knees up to her chest, she can expose her vagina for deeper penetration. He is able to caress her breasts and she can reach back to stimulate his anus and scrotum.

Clasped legs
Partners lie face-to-face in a close embrace. Depth of penetration is increased if the man raises his upper leg slightly.

Move your leg up and down to change the depth of penetration

'Spoons' *Maximum skin contact and the fact that the man can freely caress his partner's breasts and genital area make for increased intimacy.*

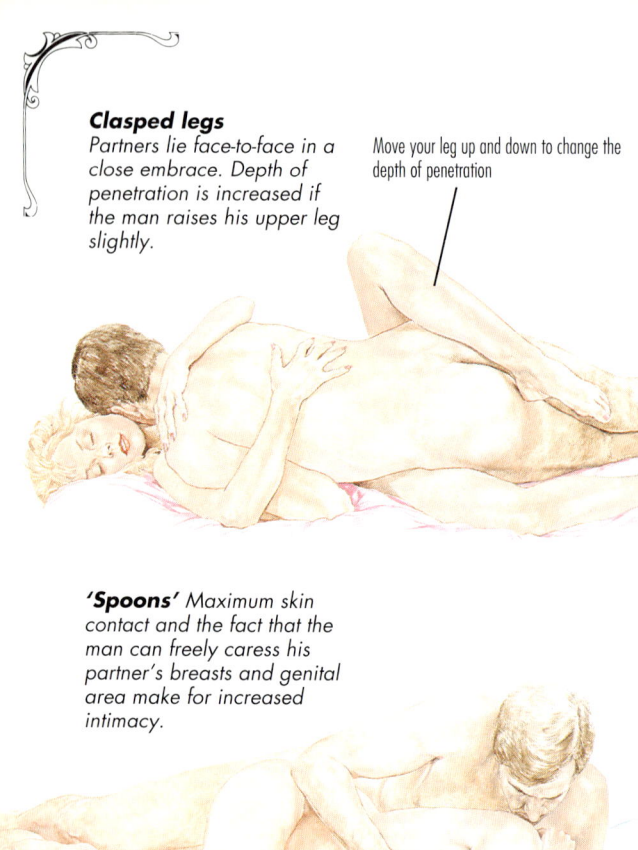

SITTING

Sex in a sitting position does not provide intense stimulation, so is a slower way to reach orgasm. Satisfaction is achieved at a leisurely, controlled pace.

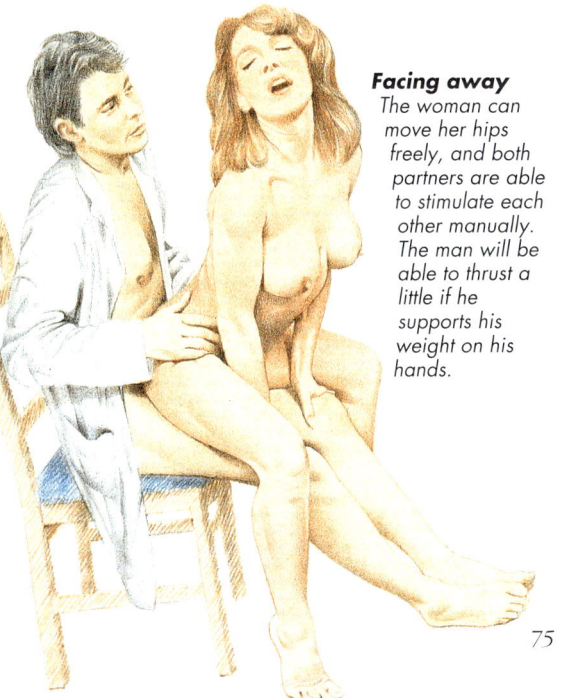

Facing away
The woman can move her hips freely, and both partners are able to stimulate each other manually. The man will be able to thrust a little if he supports his weight on his hands.

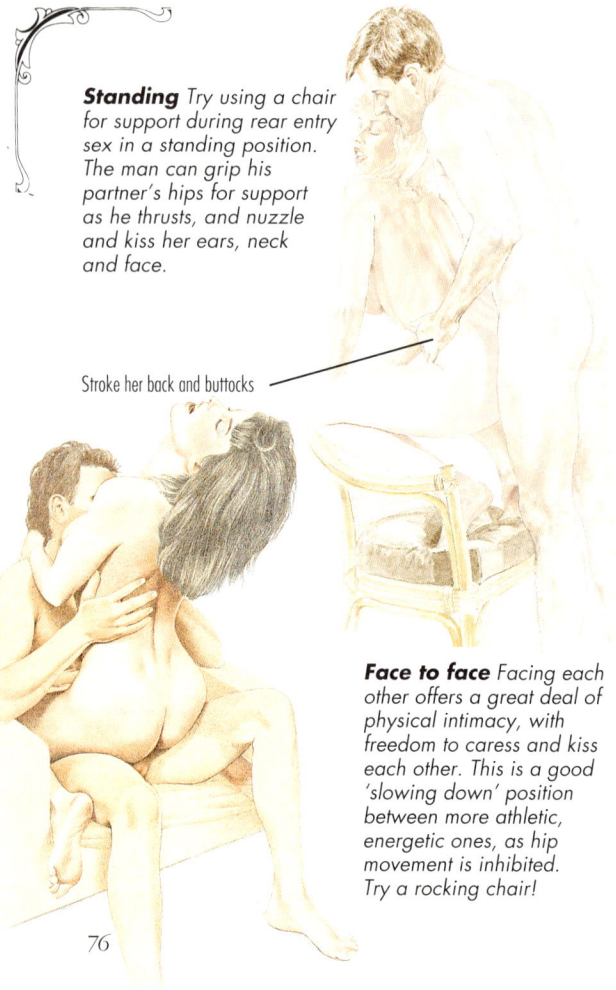

Standing Try using a chair for support during rear entry sex in a standing position. The man can grip his partner's hips for support as he thrusts, and nuzzle and kiss her ears, neck and face.

Stroke her back and buttocks

Face to face Facing each other offers a great deal of physical intimacy, with freedom to caress and kiss each other. This is a good 'slowing down' position between more athletic, energetic ones, as hip movement is inhibited. Try a rocking chair!

STANDING

Standing positions are wonderful for spontaneous lovemaking where time and space are limited.

Face to face
Particularly successful if partners are of similar height. Although the depth of penetration is limited, the woman can get more clitoral arousal, and there is more body contact for erotic foreplay.

Bend your knees if you are taller than your partner

Stand on tip-toe if you are shorter than your partner

Full lift

For the physically strong, and not suggested for the heavily pregnant woman. As the man supports his partner by holding onto her buttocks, she can grasp him snugly with her legs and pull herself up with her arms around his shoulders. Using a wall or tree for added support frees him for more relaxed thrusting.

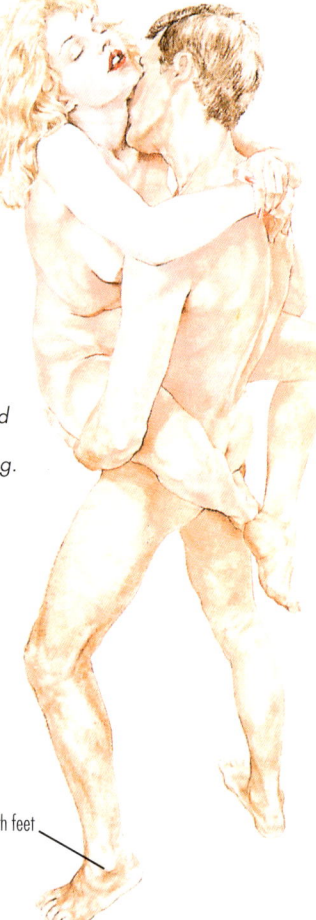

Balance the weight between both feet

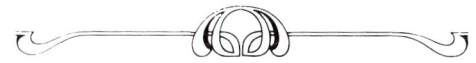

chapter five

GAMES & EROTIC TOYS

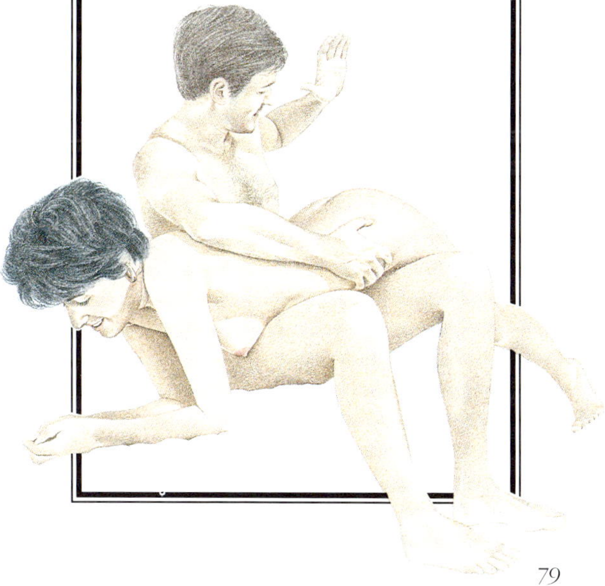

BONDAGE AND SPANKING

Games can be erotically rewarding as foreplay, and keep lovemaking from becoming routine. The only rule is that both partners are willing – pain or fear is not sexy.

Gentle restraint gives one partner permission to be passive, the other to be sexually assertive and provocative. Tie your partner's wrists with soft scarves or ties and make slow, teasing masturbation a delicious agony!

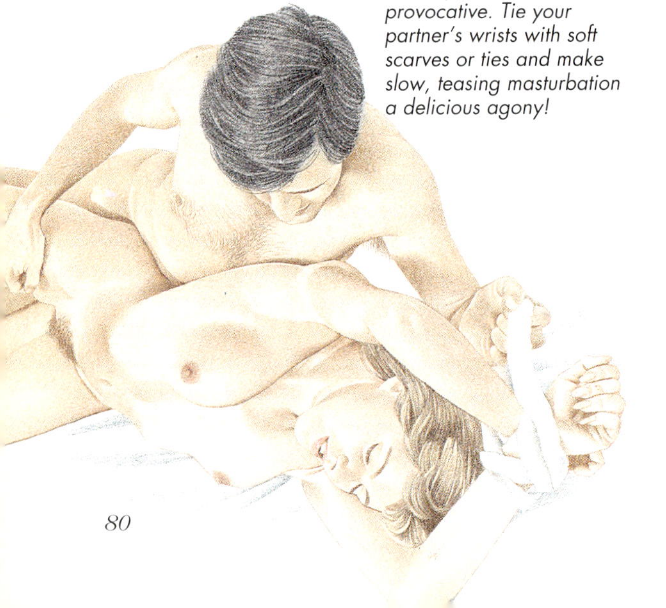

Spanking stimulates the skin, and for many is a symbol of punishment that is extremely arousing. Fantasy and role play can be put to good use by both partners, but, as with all sex games, your actions should not involve giving or receiving real pain.

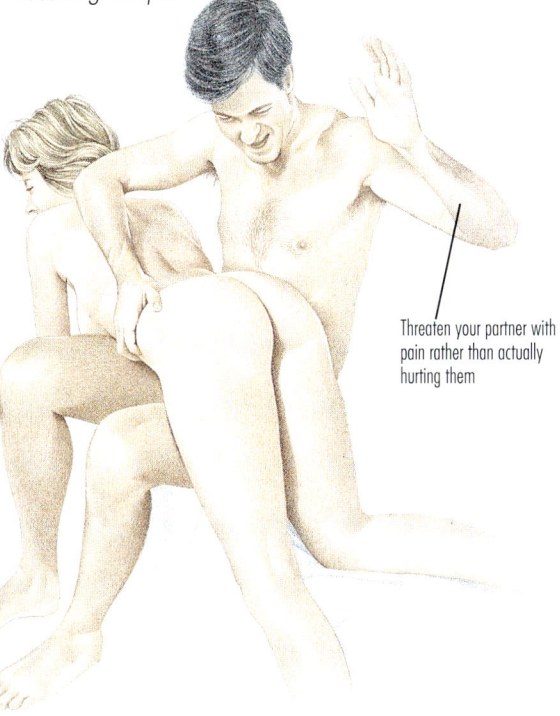

Threaten your partner with pain rather than actually hurting them

FANTASY AND ROLE PLAY

Fantasies – communicated to your partner so he or she can join in, or else kept private – are an enjoyable and erotic part of lovemaking. Your mind is your biggest erogenous zone.

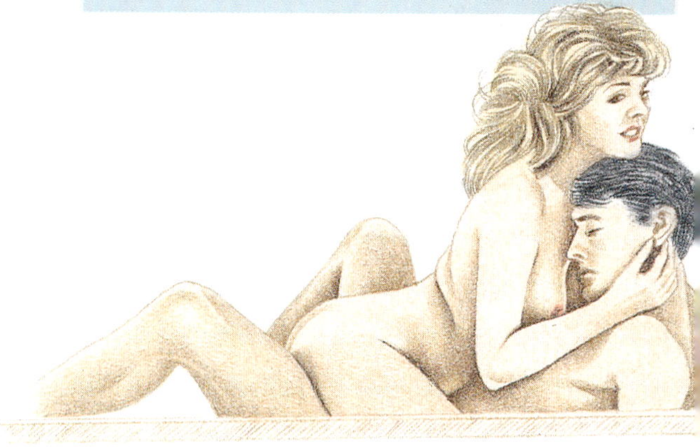

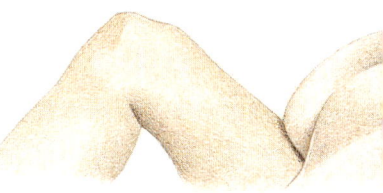

Mirrors transform sex into theatre – it is arousingly dangerous to be a voyeur, yet comfortably safe to know that you still have privacy. Many people are excited by watching themselves masturbate or make love, either naked or clothed. Fantasies can be acted out so that both the participant and the audience – ie both partners – get erotic reward.

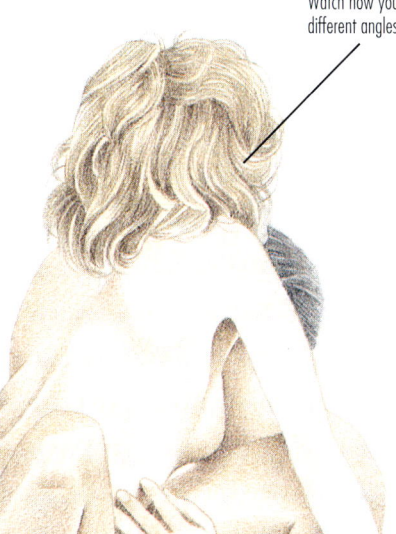

Watch how your bodies move from different angles

Dressing up to create moods and 'scenes' can make sexy games more realistic, and so more exciting for you both. Learn what turns your partner on, and what you feel seductive in, inspiring role-playing to release fantasies.

Sexy underwear, erotic for both men and women, emphasises her breasts and cleavage, and draws attention to a small waist, rounded hips and buttocks, and long legs. For him, a broad back and shoulders, strong chest and arms, lean hips, and something sizeable in his pants can be emphasized with the right clothes.

Make your legs look longer with high heels

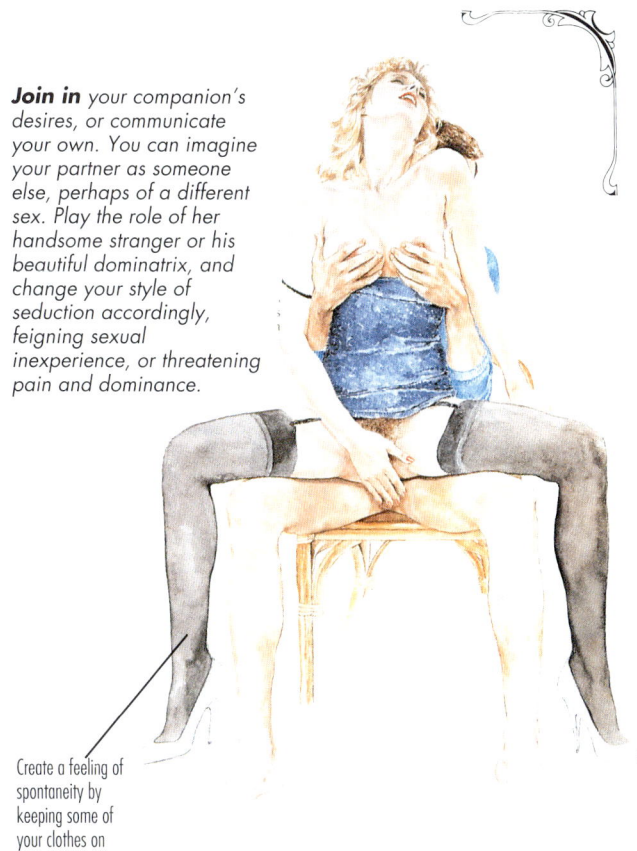

Join in your companion's desires, or communicate your own. You can imagine your partner as someone else, perhaps of a different sex. Play the role of her handsome stranger or his beautiful dominatrix, and change your style of seduction accordingly, feigning sexual inexperience, or threatening pain and dominance.

Create a feeling of spontaneity by keeping some of your clothes on

QUICKIE SEX

Short and sweet sex has the double thrill of urgent desire and the possibility of being caught. Give in to the mutual temptation – with a touch of discretion!

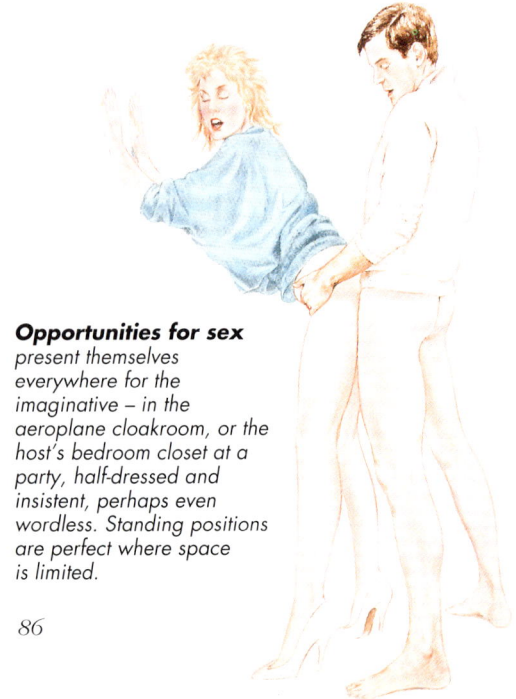

Opportunities for sex present themselves everywhere for the imaginative – in the aeroplane cloakroom, or the host's bedroom closet at a party, half-dressed and insistent, perhaps even wordless. Standing positions are perfect where space is limited.

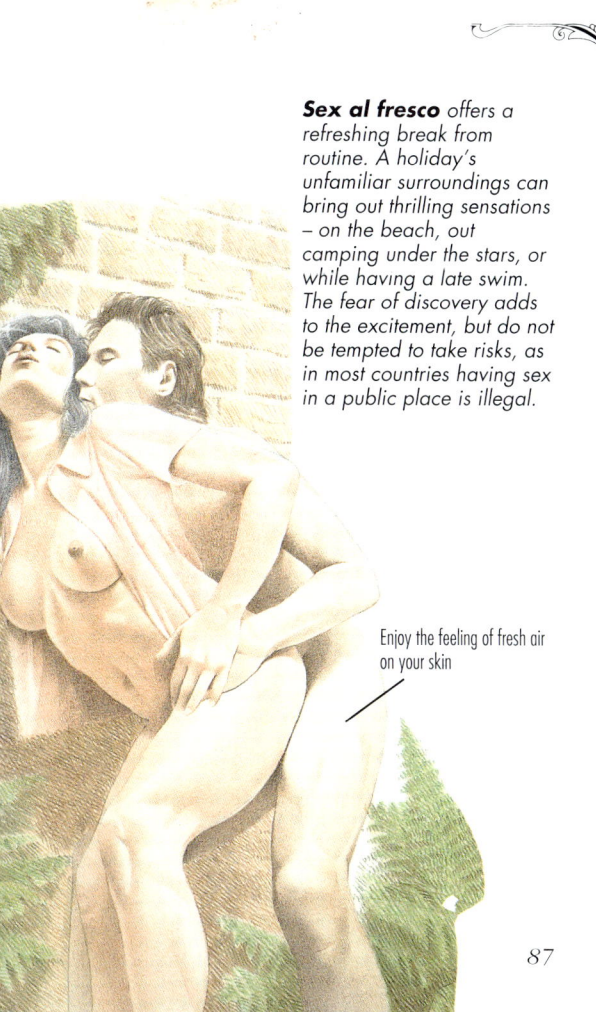

Sex al fresco offers a refreshing break from routine. A holiday's unfamiliar surroundings can bring out thrilling sensations – on the beach, out camping under the stars, or while having a late swim. The fear of discovery adds to the excitement, but do not be tempted to take risks, as in most countries having sex in a public place is illegal.

Enjoy the feeling of fresh air on your skin

SEX TOYS

The wide range of gadgets available – from vibrators and clitoral knobs to penis rings and ribbed condoms – should be used with a sense of humour, and a sense of occasion.

Vibrators can trigger intense orgasms, and can give hours of sensual pleasure. They are enjoyable for private masturbation sessions, as well as sex-play with your lover. They can be used almost everywhere, including a man's scrotum and anus, as well as a woman's genitals, anus and breasts.

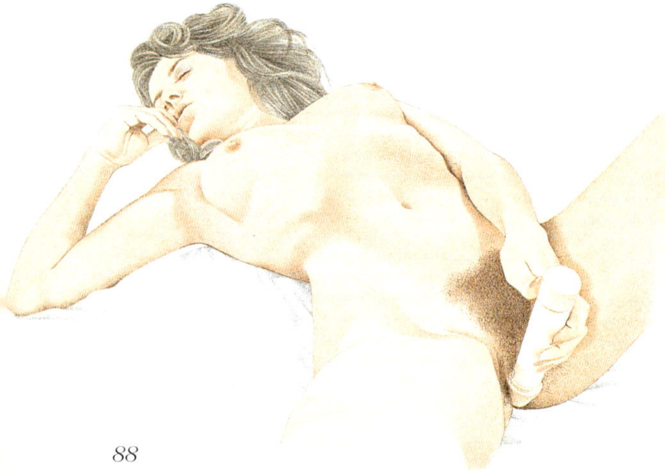

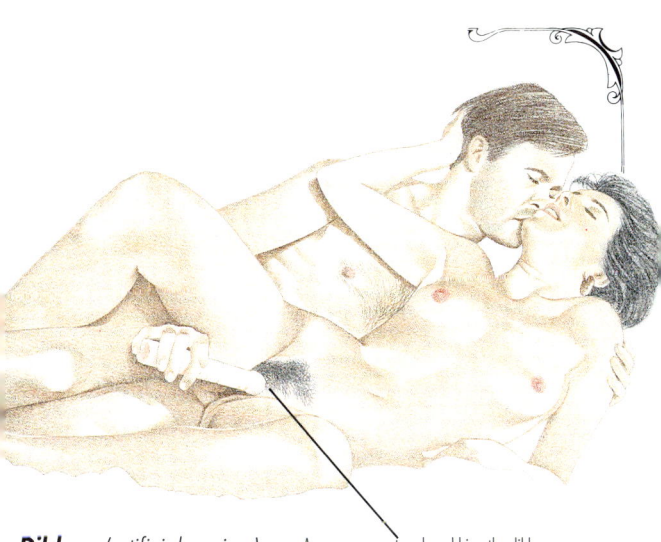

Dildoes (artificial penises) are often more visually arousing to a man, when used on his partner, than they are physically to a woman. Most women climax through stimulation of their clitoris rather than their vagina, so unless she prefers a lot of thrusting a dildo will not bring her to orgasm. Digital stimulation of the front wall of the vagina, where the ultra-sensitive G-spot is situated, will be more effective.

Arouse your partner by rubbing the dildo against her clitoris, so that the vagina is lubricated before insertion

Penile rings can help prolong erections, but should be used with care. Some are battery-operated, with a mini-vibrator attached for additional stimulation of the scrotum and anus. Watch your partner while you are arousing them them – visual stimulation can be as rewarding to you as the physical stimulation is to them. Reading and watching erotica together can also encourage a sexy mood. Soft-core videos (homemade with you two as the stars, or shop-rented) can be very arousing.

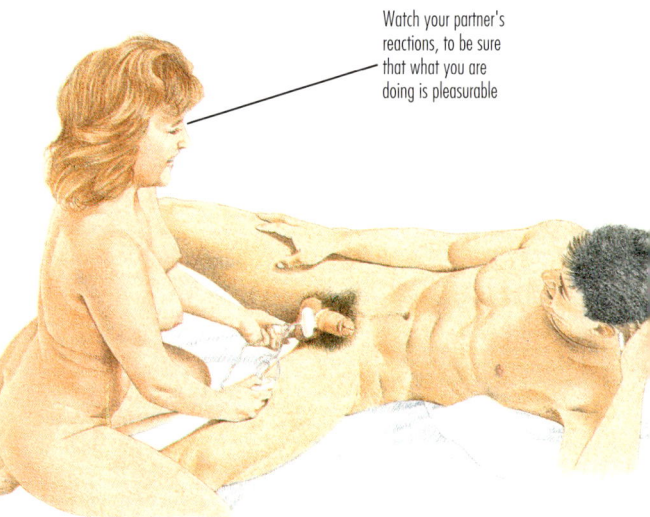

Watch your partner's reactions, to be sure that what you are doing is pleasurable

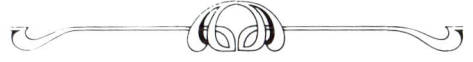

chapter six

AFTERPLAY

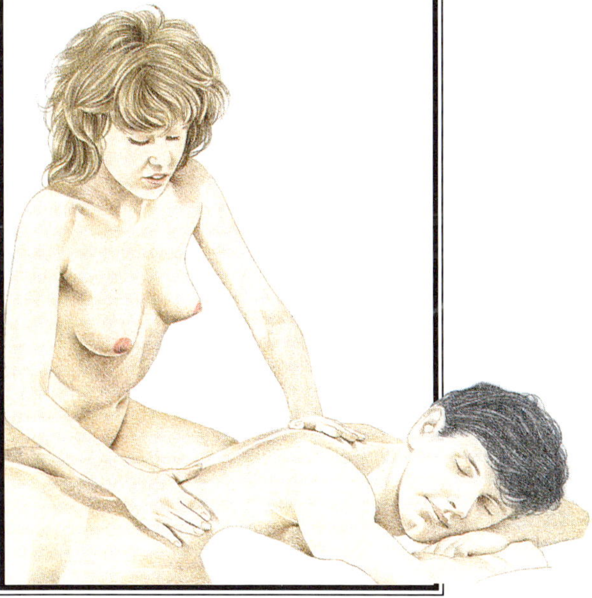

WINDING DOWN

Afterplay is every bit as important as fore- and during-play! After the fireworks, it is a time for closeness, for affection, for sharing the afterglow. It can be the most intimate time of all.

Gentle massage is an especially tender way of winding down after making love. All tension will have been released and your muscles will be especially relaxed. Try running a bath before you make love, ready to enjoy a long post-orgasmic soak with your partner.

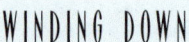

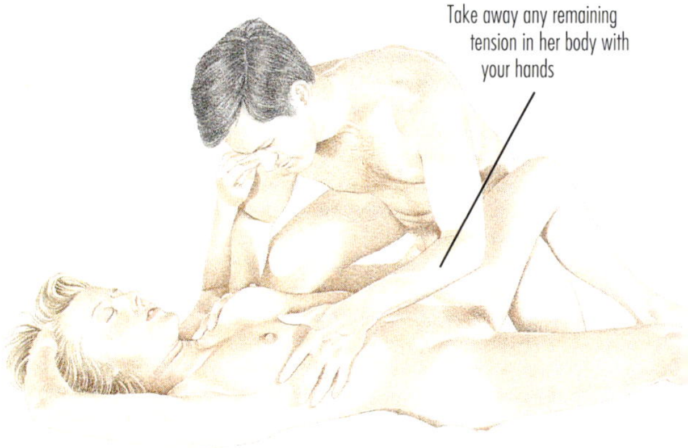

Take away any remaining tension in her body with your hands

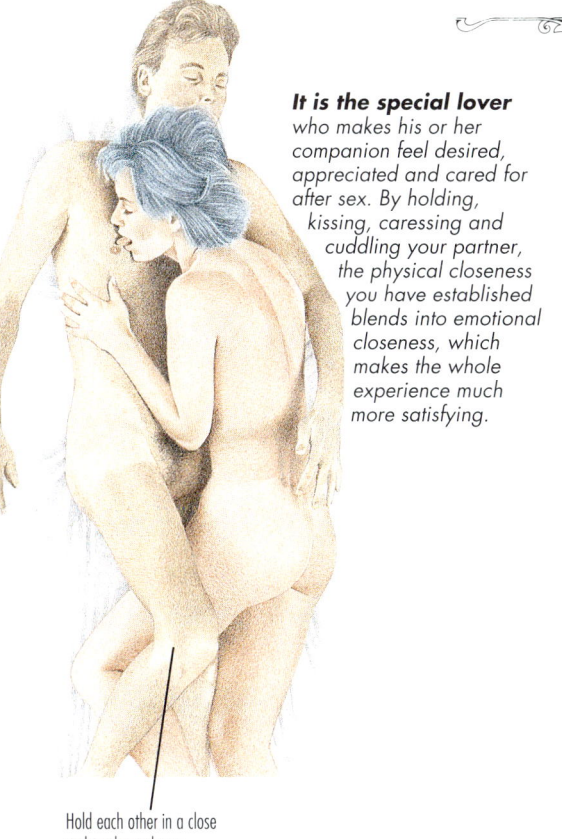

It is the special lover who makes his or her companion feel desired, appreciated and cared for after sex. By holding, kissing, caressing and cuddling your partner, the physical closeness you have established blends into emotional closeness, which makes the whole experience much more satisfying.

Hold each other in a close and tender embrace

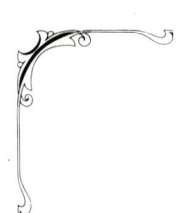

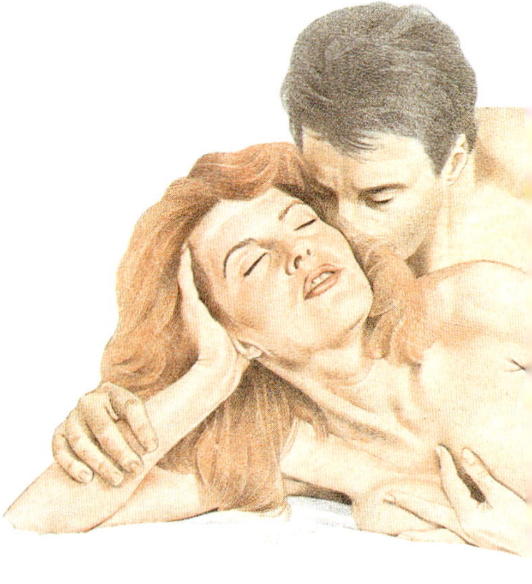

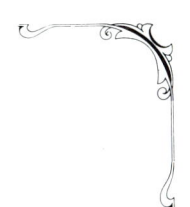

A time to talk While it is tempting, try not to roll over and fall asleep – unless you both want to, and in each other's arms. Now is the time for affectionate and playful conversation – you might even end up making love again!

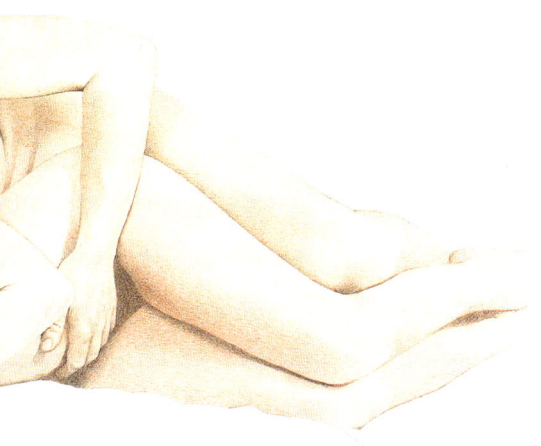

INDEX

'69' position 55
afterplay 91–5
al fresco sex 87

back 49
baths 18
bondage 80
breasts 42, 44

chest, men 46
climax see orgasms
communication 24–6, 95
condoms 11
conversation 13, 95
'crossed swords' 66
cunnilingus 54

dildoes 89
'doggy' 70
dressing up 84

erogenous zones 42–50
erotic toys 79–90
exercise 10

facing away positions
  'parting of the waves'
    64
  rear entry 68–71, 76
  sitting 75
  woman dominant 57
fantasy 82–5
feet 48
fellatio 52
females see women
food 19
foreplay 27–50
French kissing 29
'frog' 61

games 79–90

Kegel exercises 16
kissing 28–9
kneeling position 60

location 23–4

male
  masturbation 37, 39
  orgasm 14
man dominant positions
  62–7
  'crossed swords' 66
  feet on shoulders 63
  hips lifted 67
  missionary position 62
  'parting of the waves'
    64
  press-ups 65
massage 13, 20–1, 92
masturbation 36–41
mirrors 83
missionary position 62

neck 49
nipples 44–5, 46
non-verbal expression 26

opportunities 86
oral sex 13, 52–5
orgasms 14–16

'parting of the waves'
  64
penile rings 90
performance 51–78
positions 51–78
press-ups 65

'quickie' sex 86

rear entry 68–71
  'doggy' 70
  lying flat 68, 71
  side-by-side 73
  sitting 69, 75
  standing 76
reverse missionary 57
role play 82–5

'scissors' 59
self-confidence 12
sexually transmitted
  diseases (STDs) 11, 13

showers 18
side-by-side positions
  72–4
  clasped legs 74
  legs raised 72
  man behind 73
  'spoons' 74
sitting positions 75–6
  face to face 66, 76
  rear entry 69, 75
  woman dominant 57,
    58
skin 50
'soixante-neuf' 55
spanking 81
'spoons' 74
standing positions 77–8
  face to face 77
  full lift 78
  rear entry 71, 76

teasing 21
thighs 33, 47
toes 48
tonguing 32–3
touching 30–1
toys 88–90
trust 25

underwear 84
undressing 34–5

vibrators 13, 88

woman dominant
  positions 56–61
  facing away 57
  'frog' 61
  on knees 60
  lying flat 68
  reverse missionary 57
  'scissors' 59
  sitting up 58
women
  masturbation 36–7,
    38
  orgasm 14